Teaching Primary Care Nursing

L. Colette Jones, R.N., Ph.D., certified nurse-practitioner, received her diploma in nursing from Minneapolis General Hospital School of Nursing, a Bachelor of Science degree in nursing from the University of Nebraska, a Master's degree in maternal-infant nursing from the Catholic University of America, and a doctoral degree in human development education from the University of Maryland. She also received a certificate as an adult nurse practitioner from the University of Maryland School of Nursing and is certified as an adult nurse practitioner by the American Nurses' Association. She has been on the faculty of the University of Maryland School of Nursing, teaching both undergraduate and graduate courses since 1972. She is currently an associate professor in the graduate primary care nursing program. In addition to teaching, she conducts research in family nursing with emphasis on the father-infant relationship and on the nurse practitioner role. Dr. Jones has written several research and clinical articles and book chapters. She has also written and managed training grants funding primary care programs. Dr. Jones has maintained a part-time practice as a nurse practitioner in family, college, and adult health care settings.

TEACHING PRIMARY CARE NURSING

Concepts and Curriculum for Expanded Roles

L. Colette Jones, R.N., Ph.D., C.-A.N.P.

Springer Publishing Company/New York

Springer Publishing Company, Inc.
200 Park Avenue South
New York, New York 10003

84 85 86 87 88 / 10 9 8 7 6 5 4 3 2 1

Library of Congress Cataloging in Publication Data

Jones, L. Colette.
  Teaching primary care nursing.
  (Springer series on the teaching of nursing ; v. 9)
  Includes bibliographies and index.
  1. Nursing—Study and teaching. 2. Nurse practitioners. I. Title. II. Series.
  [DNLM: 1. Primary Nursing Care. 2. Education, Nursing. 3. Curriculum.
  W1 SP685SG v.9 / WY 18 J773t]
RT71.J76 1984   610.73'07'1173   84-1222
ISBN 0-8261-3930-2

Printed in the United States of America

*To my family who told me I could,
and to my students who told me I should—
I write this book.*

Contents

APPENDIXES

Contributors

Thomasine D. Guberski, R.N., M.S., C.-A.N.P., Assistant Professor, Primary Care Programs, University of Maryland School of Nursing, Baltimore, Maryland

Mary Fry Rapson, R.N., Ph.D., C.-A.N.P., Chairperson, Junior Year, Undergraduate Studies, University of Maryland School of Nursing, Baltimore, Maryland

Marilyn Winterton Edmunds, R.N., M.S., C.-A.N.P., Assistant Professor, Primary Care Programs, University of Maryland School of Nursing, Baltimore, Maryland

Preface and Acknowledgments

In the few short years since the first nurse practitioner program began, the planners and instructors have held fast to the vision of an expanded role within nursing. Our efforts to prepare a nurse who could meet the primary health care needs of underserved areas have been largely successful. Even as a surplus of physicians is predicted, many consumers—not just in underserved areas—discovered that they received not only adequate, but superior, health care from a nurse practitioner. The strong emphasis in nursing on health promotion and disease prevention combined with the increased need for chronic illness care has made the nurse practitioner a nurse for all seasons. A hardy, pioneer lot from the beginning, we are moving the challenge into the halls of academe in master's and doctoral programs and are engaging in sophisticated campaigns to market our considerable talents.

The purpose of this book is to bring together the essence of program planning, curriculum development, instructional methods, and the particular content required in a nurse practitioner program. Much of the material can also apply to the teaching of assessment skills and primary care content on the bachelor's level. As the nurse practitioner moves into the mainstream of nursing, many continuing education short courses are closing or moving into master's programs. However, many strong programs continue and may for some time.

Content in this book can be used in those programs if attention is paid to the background of entering students. However, I want to make it clear that I support the movement of nurse practitioner programs to master's programs because of the synthesis of nursing and medical knowledge required and the complex role that many practitioners must shape for themselves.

Part I of the book discusses those issues and problems bearing on the role of the nurse practitioner, including the application of nursing theory to that role. Part II is the core of the book and addresses program development, curriculum sequencing, and instructional materials and methods. Special emphasis is placed on planning clinical experiences for students. Part III covers research and evaluation of programs. As the educational dollar shrinks, this will become an even more important faculty function.

I want to acknowledge the help of many colleagues who reviewed one or more chapters at various stages of completion. They are: Beverly Baldwin, Judith Court, Marilyn Edmunds, Hurdis Griffith, Cynthia Northrup, Judith Ryan, Norma Small, and Carolyn Waltz. In addition, Dolores Stewart typed the manuscript several times over with great patience and accuracy.

L.C.J.

Introduction

When a new role in nursing—or any other practice profession—emerges, educators must also be developed to teach the new "breed." It is no easy matter to learn new content, skills, and role behavior and then, almost simultaneously, begin teaching it to others. The process becomes of necessity that of "each one teach one" for a period of time.

In the nearly twenty years of the nurse practitioner movement, nursing education has played this kind of catch-up. Many teachers have come with clinical preparation in other fields and taken a nurse practitioner continuing education course while teaching in another area. Many have never worked extensively in the nurse practitioner role. At the same time we now have nurse practitioners with several years clinical experience but no preparation in nursing education.

The following chapters are designed to help potential educators of nurse practitioners regardless of prior experience as they become prepared to teach in a nurse practitioner program or teach segments of the skills and role to students at any level of preparation.

It will be helpful to define a few confusing terms that are used throughout the book.

• *Nurse Practitioner.* A professional nurse who has completed a formal educational program, either master's or continuing education, to prepare for an expanded role in nursing as a nurse practitioner. The nurse practitioner provides comprehensive direct care including assessment, diagnosis, and treatment of illness and health maintenance to individuals, families, and groups in a variety of settings including clinics, homes, offices, industry, schools, and other institutions. Most nurse practitioners are prepared to give care to a defined population, for example, adults, children, women, families, college students.

• *Primary Care.* Primary care has two dimensions: (1) care of individuals at first contact with the health care system; and (2) continuity of care for health maintenance, management of illness, and referral to other providers over time.

• *Expanded Role.* The assumption of new roles and functions beyond the traditional role. Usually includes greater responsibility, autonomy, and accountability in management of patient care for a given population. Functions may overlap with medicine and/or other health care providers.

It is important to note that although most nurse practitioners today deliver primary care, and this book is aimed at teachers of primary care nurse practitioners, the two terms are not forever wedded. In fact, nurse practitioners already are working in institutions that provide acute, chronic, and extended care. It is possible that the term nurse practitioner may eventually connote a more independent decision-making role with functions that vary according to the setting. For instance, many nurse practitioners now work in acute care hospitals doing initial assessments and working with others to provide continuing care throughout the hospital stay. Others are in nursing homes and rehabilitation centers, essentially providing tertiary care. It behooves nursing educators to monitor and guide such trends so that educational programs meet the needs of students and the reality of practice.

I
Foundations of
Primary Care Nursing

1

Theory and Primary Care Nursing

Whether or not we are aware of it, primary care nurse practitioners and educators hold beliefs and values that influence our practice. These beliefs concern human nature, health, nursing, the environment, and our expanded role in nursing. In addition, we have beliefs about students and learning that guide our teaching. The combination of beliefs about nursing and education are expressed in the selection of curriculum content and instructional methods.

One's philosophy of nursing expressed in beliefs and values is, in reality, one's theory of nursing. Hence, all nurses do practice and teach using one or more theories, conceptual frameworks, or constructs. It is important for instructors in primary care nursing to examine these beliefs and values about both nursing and education, because they are transferred to students implicitly, if not explicitly, in the process of teaching. Without some organized thinking and planning, the messages conveyed to students can be confusing.

The purpose of this chapter is to offer some guidelines by which theories can be evaluated for use in primary care nursing education. Some of the major theorists are examined using the criteria.

DEFINITIONS

Much time can be spent in debating whether a set of beliefs constitutes a theory, a conceptual framework, or a model. Some authors only label as theory those sets of beliefs that are very comprehensive

3

or grand. For them, lesser theoretical statements are conceptual frameworks. In this chapter, the term theory is interpreted to mean "a statement that purports to account for or characterize some phenomenon" (Stevens, 1979, p. 1).

A theory identifies the salient elements of a phenomenon, then proposes some relationships among those elements. A theory is, in some ways, a symbolic representation of a concept like a road map. The elements in a theory are concepts of varying complexity and abstraction. A concept is a word that brings forth mental images of the properties of things. Concepts may be concrete in nature such as "table" or "bed" or more abstract such as "love" or "health." In nursing theories, the salient concepts are more often complex and abstract. The concepts of nursing, humanity, society, patient, and health. are some that are most commonly included.

Theories can be divided into those that are descriptive and those that are explanatory or predictive. The descriptive theory only identifies salient elements or concepts of a phenomenon. A theory of health care that defines the concepts of nurse, physician, and patient is a descriptive theory. Explanatory theories go a step further and predict or explain why and how the elements relate to each other. If a theory about health care states how the nurse relates to the physician and patient, it becomes explanatory or predictive. An "if-then" relationship can be formulated from a predictive theory. For example, a theory that states that the nurse can manipulate the environment to improve health could be operationalized by stating that if a nurse practitioner improves the air quality of a work environment, the health of employees will improve. Although prediction is a higher level, descriptive theories are important in delineating what elements "belong" in a phenomenon.

PRIMARY CARE NURSING AND THEORIES

Primary care nursing is concerned with both descriptive and predictive theories. Descriptive theories are important in that they define the major elements of a phenomenon. In a new field such as primary care, it is to be expected that theory might be at the descriptive level. A theory for nursing that does not include concepts such as diagnosis, illness, collaboration, or similar concepts, does not include expanded role functions as they are now defined. Indeed, this is the logic used by critics of the nurse practitioner role who say that it is not within the province of nursing. Curriculum builders of expanded role programs act "as if" the role were within nursing and therefore should not embrace a restrictive theory for nursing that excludes them. Additionally, it is undoubtedly more useful to adopt middle-range theories that have a focus on realities of practice than to search for a grand theory.

Explanatory theories are of even more importance to teachers of primary care nursing because the role is relatively new and includes concepts common to other health providers as well as those accepted in nursing. Practitioners in a new role need theories that will describe, explain, and predict relationships among the new as well as the more familiar concepts of nursing. A theory that makes statements about the relationships of certain elements (i.e., nurse, physician, patient, health, illness, family) is consonant with the expanded role. At least, a theory should be chosen that does not restrict nursing in expanded roles.

For providing patient care, theories must predict the result of an interaction between nurse and patient. For instance, a theory that implicitly or explicitly says that nurses may intervene to help a patient become healthier speaks to the essence of primary care.

THEORIES FOR PRACTICE

The difficulty in selecting an existing nursing theory for primary care practice is that most describe nursing as the theorist would like it to be, not as it is. It is the author's opinion that no existing theory speaks adequately to the reality of practice in the expanded role. However, parts of several theories considered later do speak to some elements and relationships in expanded role nursing. Yet, as Stevens states, "Theory arises out of practice and once validated, returns to direct and explain that practice" (1979, p. 82).

A further consideration is the borrowing of theory from other disciplines. For instance, truths about human beings and health may be borrowed from psychology, sociology, or physiology. Borrowed theory in nursing often is redefined in nursing's image. In other words, elements and relationships take on new meaning for the discipline. An example is the application of general systems theory where words such as input, output, and negentropy have unique meanings in nursing. Theory from medicine is often adapted and integrated into nursing and the converse is true. Stevens (1979) states that borrowed theory should no longer be considered borrowed but becomes a part of nursing theory. Nursing theorists have frequently borrowed theory to define elements of their relationships. For instance, again referring to systems theory, it has provided a framework for the analysis of relationships among human beings, nursing, and the environment.

EDUCATION AND PRIMARY CARE

Nurse educators who have formal training in curriculum development and instructional methods are exposed to education theories. Some of these are mentioned in Part II. Frequently these theories are applied to the nurse-patient interaction. This is legitimate to some extent in that there are certainly parallels in the nurse-patient and teacher-learner situations. However, theories borrowed from education and applied to nursing practice often do not include the elements necessary to describe the phenomenon of primary care nursing. They may not include the patient's family and other health professions or the concept of health or illness. Teaching in areas related to health and illness may call for different elements and relationships between teacher (nurse) and learner (patient) than does classroom teaching.

EDUCATION AND NURSING THEORIES

When designing a program and the consequent curriculum there is an interplay between the chosen nursing theory and educational theory. Nursing theory becomes both content and an organizing framework for the curriculum which is planned and taught using educational theory. The sequence is usually to introduce the nursing framework early in the program to provide a particular view of patients and health care. This is akin to choosing the spot from which to take a photograph. Once the nursing theory is introduced, it can be used as an organizing theme.

Whether all courses and content areas must be taught from the viewpoint of the chosen theory is a decision faculty must make. Some supporting courses such as physiology or health care organizations might be better taught using non-nursing theories. The time that is allotted to teaching theory is another decision. In a baccalaureate program, nursing theory should determine the student's initial view of nursing. In a continuing education certificate course, students will come with some practice and possibly a theory from previous education. Here theory must be thoroughly integrated or it is meaningless in a curriculum taught over a few months. A master's program may choose to introduce several theories or only one. Master's students are able to examine theories in greater detail in several courses and to test them in practice and in thesis research. Teaching only one theory for nursing in a graduate program may narrow rather than broaden the students' philosophical base.

The interplay of nursing and educational theories comes in the curriculum building beyond the introduction of the nursing theory. Courses may be organized around elements such as nursing systems or around particular relationships such as the "patient in his family" theme. The choice of content and sequencing is based on sound educational theory. For instance, teaching may use a theme of simple to complex issues such as individual-family-community or common problems to less common problems. There is not always a perfect fit of curriculum building to educational theory because pragmatic concerns such as the numbers in a clinical site intervene. Additionally, there may be different opinions about sequencing that must be resolved. If a health-illness continuum is an organizing theme, is it really easier to teach and learn about health than about illness or is it complex but necessary information to proceed to learning about illness? Perhaps health is a more complex concept than illness. Faculty must make some initial decisions but be ready to modify them if future evaluation shows a need for change.

Many nursing theories have been developed by educators rather than by practitioners of nursing. Moreover, they project what the theorists believe nursing should be and not what it is. No wonder that nurse practitioners who believe their practice is within the scope of nursing find existing theories inadequate or contrary to their beliefs. For instance, most nursing theories do not deal adequately with the management of total health care by nurses, nor do they speak to the complexities of the health care team.

CRITERIA FOR EVALUATING NURSING THEORIES

Faculty may be developing a new program within a school of nursing that has a theoretical or conceptual framework. Or they may be able to choose one for a new program. How should theories be chosen for use in a nurse practitioner or other expanded role program? One solution is to construct one's own theory, and some programs have done just that. The faculty must examine their beliefs, define elements, and cogitate about the relationships among the elements. This requires time and expertise in theory development, and consultants are usually needed to help in the process.

An alternative is to adopt one or more existing nursing theories. Pragmatically, this occurs when one or more faculty members have come from schools where they have been immersed in a specific theory. Whether or not it is the best theoretical base for expanded roles should be considered.

The focus of the remainder of this chapter is to examine some well-known nursing theories in light of their application to expanded roles. Many criteria have been proposed for evaluating theory, both internally and externally. Clarity, consistency, and logical development are considerations when looking at the internal construction of a theory. In addition, theory must be examined for relationships to the real world. This process of external criticism includes evaluating for adequacy, utility, significance, and capacity for discrimination (Stevens, 1979).

Elements of both internal and external criticism will be used here as the specific theories are discussed. Questions which can be addressed by the reader are listed below. Others may be addressed for specific program needs and the reader is referred to the suggested readings at the end of the chapter for other viewpoints on theory analysis.

• *Scope.* What is the scope of the theory? Does it contain the necessary elements? Is it adequate for nursing in expanded roles? Is it a grand or middle-range theory?

• *Complexity.* How *complex* is the theory? Is it appropriate for the level of practice? Is it too complex for students to learn and begin to apply in practice in the allotted time?

• *Values.* What values or biases are implicit and explicit? Are they compatible with the faculty's view of the expanded role? (Values may be derived from stated assumptions or premises.)

• *Discrimination.* Does the theory differentiate the boundaries of nursing practice from those of other health professions? Does it address or admit overlapping boundaries?

• *Utility.* How useful is the theory for nursing practice? Will it provide the student (or practitioner) with a frame of reference from which to view practice in the settings for which the program prepares graduates?

• *Testability.* How *testable* is the theory in practice? For instance, can a researcher compare roles and relationships defined in the theory with those in practice? Can a practitioner derive an if-then statement that can be applied to nursing in various situations?

• *Terminology.* Is the terminology understandable only in nursing or can it be used meaningfully in interprofessional practice? Will it help a nurse practitioner communicate to others or is it unnecessarily obscure?

SELECTED THEORIES

A few of the most commonly known theories will be discussed in relation to their use in primary care nursing practice. The same process can be used in evaluating other theories or even so-called curriculum threads or concepts. The theories that will be examined are Orem's concept of self-care agency, general systems theory, Rogers' theory of unitary man, Roy's adaptation model, and King's nursing theory. A brief synopsis (with apologies to their devotees) is followed by the author's beliefs about their application to primary care nursing.

OREM'S THEORY OF SELF-CARE

The key concept in Orem's theory is self-care, defined as those activities that individuals initiate and perform for themselves in maintaining life, health, and well-being. The ability to do this, in response to demands, reflects the person's power of agency. Two categories of self-care demands have been identified: universal self-care and health deviation self-care. The universal category contains six subcategories:

- air, water, and food
- excrements
- activity and rest
- solitude and social interaction
- hazards to life and well-being
- being normal

Those self-care demands in health deviations are disease-derived and medically-derived (demands due to diagnosis or treatment) (Coleman, 1980, pp. 315–316).

In this theory, nursing is caring for, assisting with, or doing something for the patient to achieve self-care. Basically, the nurse intervenes only when the patient has a deficit in self-care and a need for nursing care can be established. Orem identified three steps in the nursing process: (1) assessment and diagnosis; (2) designing and planning systems of nursing care; and (3) providing and controlling the delivery of nursing assistance.

Further, three basic designs of nursing are elaborated: (1) wholly compensatory; (2) supportive-educative; and (3) partly compensatory. A method of classifying patients according to nursing situations is also detailed (Coleman, 1980, pp. 319–320). The Orem self-care theory is being further elaborated by the Nursing Development Conference Group and tested in practice. The concept of nursing, especially, has been developed in greater detail than in initial publications. Some recent writings on Orem's theory are listed at the end of this chapter.

The biases and values of the theory are apparent in selected assumptions (Orem, 1979).

1. Self-care is a learned activity. (p. 132)
2. Each adult has the right and responsibility to care for himself. He may have responsibility for others. (p. 132)
3. Nursing is deliberative action performed by individuals on behalf of others. (p. 108)

Orem's theory, although developed by educators, has application in practice, is comprehensive, and certainly encompasses expanded roles in nursing. Diagnosis is an integral concept and the role of the practitioner is explicitly delineated in several settings (Orem, 1979, pp. 268–271). The values inherent in Orem's theory, that is, that people are free to accept or reject help, may remove many potential patients from nursing. The terminology is somewhat unique but is being assimilated into nursing literature enough that words such as self-care and agency are familiar to many nurse educators and practitioners. One of the advantages of the theory is that it is being tested by practice-oriented researchers.

In early stages, Orem did not give detailed guidelines for assessment. However, the most recent edition of *Concept Formalization in Nursing: Process and Product* (1979) elaborates on assessing the deficits in self-care.

Because this theory speaks to the nurse-patient relationships, it should be useful in a continuing education nurse practitioner program and for baccalaureate programs with an expanded role component. Earlier the level of complexity may not have been adequate for a graduate program, but the continuing development by a defined group makes it useful on all levels at which primary care nursing might be taught. The values inherent in the concepts of self-care define the nurse's role somewhat narrowly according to some critics because the patient must identify his or her own need for care.

SYSTEMS MODELS

Several nursing theories use a general systems approach, but are not truly systems theories (i.e., Rogers). The systems approach can also be used to develop a model or models to be used in a particular program.

The elements in a systems approach are the systems and subsystems one chooses to include. The systems may be biological, psychological, or sociological in nature but are always open systems. The use of the term holistic system is somewhat of an anachronism in that it is necessary to define lesser systems or elements in order to assess system functioning. However, the term is used by some theorists with the caveat that a holistic system is greater than the sum of its parts.

More than other approaches, systems-based theories speak to boundaries of the systems. In addition, they describe relationships between systems (inputs, outputs, and feedback) and what goes on within a system (processes or throughput).

The advantage of using a systems approach is that it offers a way of viewing the world that can be generalized beyond the particular nursing theory. There is no limit to the ability to apply the general model from the cellular level to personality to world health care. Each system, in essence, represents a concept of varying complexity. Essentially, general systems theory is a structure for developing theory.

In addition, values or biases determine what systems are chosen to be included and what boundaries, input, output, and throughput are proposed. For instance, a model with the family as a focal system implies a different value than one in which the patient is a system interacting with his environment which contains other individuals. Some models focus upon the person as the system and do not speak to the role (input) of the nurse. The inclusion of the person, health, nursing, and environment as systems is necessary for a comprehensive systems-based theory. Furthermore, a model of humans and their subsystems can be used to teach the physiology, pathology, and psychology content in a nurse practitioner curriculum. The inclusion of other elements in the health care system is important in theorizing about nurses in expanded roles.

As evident in the discussion above, the complexity of systems models varies. In choosing this approach, faculty must decide which elements to include that convey their philosophy of the expanded role yet is parsimonious. The reality of time allocation in teaching a model is a consideration. A continuing education program may choose a less complex but utilitarian model.

Systems models can be used to predict outcomes if the inputs, outputs, and processes are well defined. For instance, it is helpful to predict the efficacy of a nursing action (output) when the inputs and processes of the patient system are known.

The terminology of general systems theory is sometimes cumbersome when applied to nursing. Entropy, negentropy, and equilibrium were borrowed from earlier physical systems terminology and are often misused. Conversely, input and output and feedback have become commonly understood terms.

Figure 1-1 depicts some elements that could be expected in a comprehensive model applied to a primary care nurse practitioner program.

Figure 1-2 specifies some of the processes, inputs, and outputs in a portion of the larger model shown in Figure 1-1.

In any new field such as primary care, a systems model is helpful if:

1. The elements (systems) are clearly specified.
2. There is a focus on boundaries (i.e., roles and functions).

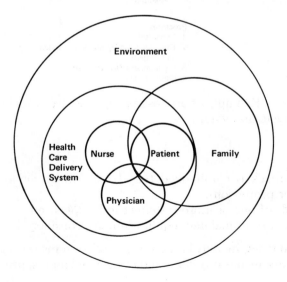

Figure 1-1. Example of a systems model

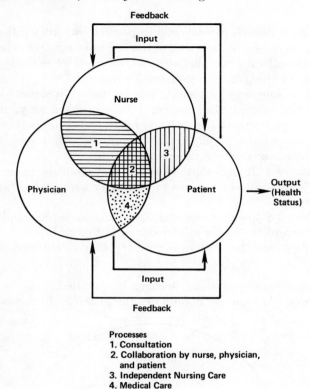

Figure 1–2.   Example of processes, input, and output in a patient/ nurse/physician system

3. Feedback is emphasized (i.e., from patient, environment, or other profession).
4. Goals of one or more systems can be specified.
5. Processes to maintain equilibrium are considered.

Existing nursing models based on general systems theory generally focus on one or more systems and on selected inputs, processes, and outputs.

ROGERS' THEORY OF UNITARY MAN

Rogers' theory focuses on unitary man. She puts forth the precept that man can only be studied as a whole. In doing so, four building blocks are important: energy fields, the universe of open systems, patterns and organization, and four-dimensionality. She states that:

> Unitary man (is) a four-dimensional energy field identified by pattern and organization and manifesting characteristics and behaviors that are different from those of the parts and which cannot be predicted from knowledge of the parts (Rogers, 1980, p. 332).

Similarly, environment is described in terms of a four-dimensional negentropic energy field.

Rogers uses the concept of homeodynamics and proposes three principles—heliacy, resonancy, and complementarity—related to the interaction between the human and environmental fields. She sees unitary man and the environment as being involved in evolution where the rate of change is accelerating. Consequently, norms of human behavior are always changing and evolving.

Although the concept of nursing is not highly developed in Roger's theory, she does state that "nursing is committed to maintaining and promoting human health and to provide evaluative, therapeutic, and rehabilitative services to people" (1970, p. 82).

Because this theory was developed by the dialectic method, it does not offer a way of analyzing or assessing man through subsystems or other parts of the whole. It also does not give specific actions nurses can take to maintain and promote health.

Rogers' theory is global and without the practice-based derivations that make a theory most useful in expanded roles. In fact, Rogers has indicated that she does not believe the expanded role is within nursing practice. "The activities commonly attributed to nursing's 'expanded role' generally replace nursing practice with non-nursing functions" (1972, p. 44). This is not to imply that all of the concepts proposed are inappropriate for primary care nurse educators. The current emphasis on holistic health care is a logical extension of the idea of unitary man. Based on a holistic approach, colleagues and former students have applied Rogers' theory in the practice setting. The concept of therapeutic touch grew out of some of Rogers' basic ideas about human beings and energy fields and forced nursing to look beyond Western medicine and nursing for therapeutic intervention (Krieger, 1981).

THE ROY ADAPTATION MODEL

The Roy Adaptation Model is a systems model that focuses on the patient as the principal system, the interaction of the patient with his or her environment, and the nurse's interaction with the patient and the environment. Eight assumptions underlie the Roy model and reveal values in the theory base:

- Assumption 1: The person is a bio-psycho-social being.
- Assumption 2: The person is in constant interaction with a changing environment.
- Assumption 3: To cope with a changing world, the person uses both innate and acquired mechanisms, which are bio-logic, psychologic, and social in origin.
- Assumption 4: Health and illness are one inevitable dimension of the person's life.
- Assumption 5: To respond positively to environmental changes, the person must adapt.
- Assumption 6: The person's adaptation is a function of the stimulus he is exposed to and his adaptation level.
- Assumption 7: The person's adaptation level is such that it comprises a zone indicating the range of stimulation that will lead to a positive response.
- Assumption 8: The person is conceptualized as having four modes of adaptation: physiologic needs, self-concept, role function, and interdependence relations (Roy, 1980, pp. 180–182).

It is evident by the assumptions that this is a practice-oriented model based on a particular view of man. The elements of man, health, and environment are present with man being the most highly developed concept in the model. Roy further states that "the nursing goal of supporting and promoting patient adaptation is important for patient welfare" (p. 183). The goal of nursing activity is promoting patient adaptation in the four modes. Some common needs in the four modes are listed in Table 1-1.

Nursing assessment is carried out on two levels, by identification of needs in each adaptive mode and by recognition of the patient's position on the health-illness continuum. The nurse then makes a diagnosis. Nursing interventions are used to manipulate influencing factors in the four modes.

Table 1–1. Basic Needs

A.   Basic Physiologic Needs

    1.   Exercise and rest
    2.   Nutrition
    3.   Elimination
    4.   Fluid and Electrolytes
    5.   Oxygen
    6.   Circulation
    7.   Regulation

        a.   Temperature
        b.   Senses
        c.   Endocrine System

B.   Self-Concept

    1.   Physical self
    2.   Personal self
    3.   Interpersonal self

C.   Role Mastery

D.   Interdependence

Note: Adapted from Conceptual Models for Nursing Practice, 2nd ed., by M. Riehl and C. Roy. New York: Appleton-Century-Crofts, 1980, pp. 185–186.

The Roy model is comprehensive and can be applied to practice. The concepts of man and health are more highly developed than that of nursing intervention. The theory has been used for curriculum development (Roy, 1973) and some practice-based research. The terminology is not esoteric and should be understandable in an interprofessional setting.

More importantly, the scope of practice implicit in the model does not exclude expanded nursing roles. In fact, the Roy model has been used as a basis for a nurse practitioner curriculum (Brower and Baker, 1976).

Nursing actions for the particular role can be spelled out for use in an expanded role program. For instance, a pediatric nurse practitioner program may emphasize different nursing actions than a geriatric program. The Roy Adaptation Model is indeed adaptable to many settings. A further advantage is the number of publications available to explicate the model and its use in different situations. See the list of suggested readings at the end of this chapter for examples.

KING'S THEORY

King's theory focuses on the interaction between patient and nurse rather than on either actor. She defines nursing as:

> a process of action, reaction, and interaction whereby nurse and client share information about their perceptions . . . identify specific goals, problems, or concerns . . . explore means to achieve a goal and agree to means to the goal (transaction). (King, 1981, p. 2)

She further states that the "domain of nursing includes promotion of health, maintenance and restoration of health, care of the sick and injured, and care of the dying" (p. 4).

Although King's theory is reportedly based on a systems model, the emphasis is on the interaction between the personal systems of nurse and patient. Two or more interacting personal systems are called interpersonal systems. The highest system level is that of social systems such as educational systems, family systems, and health care systems. Relevant concepts at each system level are identified. Concepts salient to the personal systems are perception, self, body image, growth and development, and time and space. Those identified for interpersonal systems are role, interaction, communication, transaction, and stress. Finally, those that apply to social systems are organization, power, authority, states, decision making, and role.

King's philosophical assumptions about human beings are that they are social, sentient, rational, reacting, perceiving, controlling, purposeful, action-oriented, and time-oriented. Additional assumptions about nurse-client interactions are as follows:

- Perceptions of nurse and of client influence the interaction process.
- Goals, needs, and values of nurse and client influence the interaction process.
- Individuals have a right to knowledge about themselves.
- Individuals have a right to participate in decisions that influence their life, their health, and community services.
- Health professionals have a responsibility to share information that helps individuals make informed decisions about their health care.
- Individuals have a right to accept or reject health care.
- Goals of health practitioners and goals of recipients of health care may be incongruent. (pp. 143–144)

The transaction between nurse and patient is highly valued and the most highly developed concept. Nearly all the examples given for all three levels are in hospital settings. The boundaries of nursing are not well defined except in the one-to-one patient-nurse interaction.

To be used for a comprehensive theory of practice in expanded roles, King's theory must be extended and/or interpolated. In fact, little attention is given to nursing in ambulatory settings or the relationships of nursing to other health providers. The conceptualization of the nurse-patient interaction as comprised of action, reaction, disturbance, mutual goal setting, exploring means to achieve the goal, agreeing on means, and transaction is a useful way to teach and analyze the nurse-patient relationship. The terminology is not obscure except for the confusion of the term transaction which is not used in the same way as in transactional analysis.

THE MEDICAL MODEL

The medical model as an organizing principle for curriculum development has worked well for medical educators, or it certainly would have been abandoned long ago. It has not served well in nursing as evidenced by the development of nursing theory. Many nurses in expanded roles obtain the patient's data base with a format using organ systems. This serves well in the areas of physical illness but is inadequate in assessing many of the areas of concern to nursing such as activities of daily living, and spiritual and psychological aspects of health and illness.

Some of the deficits of the medical model for assessment are in the paucity of psychological, sociological, and environmental data obtained. After analyzing man by anatomical or functional body systems, there is no attempt to resynthesize the data to provide a holistic assessment.

It is possible to supplement the medical data base to allow a more comprehensive assessment. For younger patients, especially, this involves adding substantial information on growth and development. For all age levels, additional questions about areas such as family, life style, and work environment must be asked.

Nurses in expanded roles and interdisciplinary settings will, for the foreseeable future, need to record data using the medical model to some extent. However, it can and should be supplemented to obtain sufficient data for a nursing assessment. The medical and nursing models are not mutually exclusive. Many physicians now embrace concepts previously exclusive to nursing. However, the mainstream of medicine has not yet expanded its teachings to include them.

SUMMARY

Nursing theories for primary care should be evaluated for scope, complexity, values, ability to discriminate nursing from other professions, utility, testability in practice, and for unambiguous terminology. Some existing nursing theories were summarized and commented upon for use in primary care and expanded nursing practice.

These and other theories should be examined carefully before adoption for use in an expanded role program.

If faculty wish to develop their own theories or extend an existing one, time and expert consultants are needed. Some of the essential concepts that should be addressed in a global theory for primary care nursing are:

patient (or client)	diagnosis
health behaviors	management (or treatment)
nurse	health
nurse practitioner	environment
health care team	health care
interdependence (professional)	illness care
collaboration	

Furthermore, some of the relationships among the elements should be elaborated on if a useful framework for practice is to result.

In a baccalaureate or continuing education program, theory is developed or selected by faculty, but in a graduate program concepts and their relationships can be added through student research. At the least, theses and dissertations should be planned to test parts of the theory in practice.

Education of nurse practitioners must be based upon well-delineated nursing theory. Teaching a theory for practice will focus the student's efforts on the reality of practice and clarify the role.

REFERENCES

Brower, H. T. F. & Baker, B. J. Using the adaptation model in a practitioner curriculum. *Nursing Outlook*, 1976, *24*, (11), 686–689.

Coleman, L. J. Orem's self-care concept of nursing. In J. P. Riehl and C. Roy, *Conceptual models for nursing practice*, 2nd ed. New York: Appleton-Century-Crofts, 1980.

Hazzard, M. E., & Kergin, D. An overview of systems theory. *Nursing Clinics of North America*, 1971, *6*, (3), 163–168.

Johnson, D. E. Development of theory: A requisite for nursing as a primary health profession. *Nursing Research*, 1974, *23*, (5), 372–377.

King, I. M. *A theory for nursing: Systems, concepts, process.* New York: John Wiley and Sons, 1981.

Krieger, D. *Foundations for holistic health nursing practice: The Renaissance nurse*. Philadelphia: J. B. Lippincott Company, 1981.
Orem, D. E. (Ed.). *Concept formalization in nursing: Process and product*, 2nd ed. Boston: Little, Brown and Company, 1979.
Rogers, M. E. *An introduction to the theoretical basis of nursing*. Philadelphia: F. A. Davis Company, 1970.
Rogers, M. E. Nursing: To be or not to be? *Nursing Outlook*, 1972, *20*, (1), 42–45.
Rogers, M. E. Nursing: A science of unitary man. In J. P. Riehl & C. Roy, *Conceptual models for nursing practice*, 2nd ed. New York: Appleton-Century-Crofts, 1980.
Roy, C. Adaptation: Implications for curriculum change. *Nursing Outlook*, 1973, *21*, 163–168.
Roy, C. *Introduction to nursing: An adaptation model*. Englewood Cliffs, New Jersey: Prentice-Hall, 1976.
Roy, C. The Roy adaptation model. In J. P. Riehl & C. Roy, *Conceptual models for nursing practice*, 2nd ed. New York: Appleton-Century-Crofts, 1980.
Stevens, B. J. *Nursing theory: Analysis, application, evaluation*. Boston: Little, Brown, and Company, 1979.

SUGGESTED READINGS

Chin, P. L. (Ed.). *Advances in nursing theory development*. Rockville, Maryland: Aspen Systems Corporation, 1983.
Chin, R. The utility of systems models and developmental models for practitioners. In W. G. Bennis, K. D. Benne, & R. Chin (Eds.). *The planning of change*. New York: Holt, Rinehart & Winston, 1961.
Dickoff, J. & James, P. Beliefs and values: basis for curriculum design. *Nursing Research*, 1968, *17*, 415–427.
Duffey, M. & Muhlenkamp, A. F. A framework for theory analysis. *Nursing Outlook*, 1974, *22*, (9), 570–574.
Hardy, M. E. Theories: Components, development, evaluation. *Nursing Research*, 1974, *23*, (2), 100–107.
Riehl, J. P. & Roy, C. *Conceptual models for nursing practice*, 2nd ed. New York: Appleton-Century-Crofts, 1980.
Roy, C. Adaptation: A conceptual framework for nursing. *Nursing Outlook*, 1970, *18*, 42.
Roy, C. Adaptation: A basis for nursing practice. *Nursing Outlook*, 1971, *19*, 254.

Roy, C. & Roberts, S. L. *Theory construction in nursing: An adaptation model*. Englewood Cliffs, New Jersey: Prentice-Hall, 1981.

Watson, A. B. & Mayers, M. G. *Assessment and documentation: Theories in action*. Thorofore, New Jersey: Charles B. Slack, 1981.

Webster, G., Jacox, A., & Baldwin, B. Nursing theory and the ghost of the received view. In J. C. McCloskey & H. K. Grace. *Current issues in nursing*. Boston: Blackwell Scientific Publications, 1981.

White, M. B. (Ed.). *Curriculum development from a nursing model: The crisis theory framework*. New York: Springer Publishing Company, 1983.

2

Issues for Nurses
in Expanded Roles

The education of nurses for expanded roles requires a reorientation of both students and instructors. Issues which are only peripheral to nurses in traditional roles take on new importance when viewed from an expanded role perspective. The faculty's stance on certain issues will determine, in part, the philosophy and purposes of the program. For instance, if they believe the major role of the nurse practitioner is in health education and screening for disease, the program will be influenced by that position. Certain critical issues must be examined when faculty are developing programs.

In addition to their philosophical implications some issues discussed here, such as conflict management, become cognitive content in the curriculum. Knowledge and skills gained in this area can be applied to colleagues, patients, and organizations. Other nurses are involved in conflict, but those in expanded roles have particular need for skills in resolving dissension. Other concepts can be presented with the purpose of broadening the student's perspective on professional issues. In addition, students can develop survival techniques for entering new and unexplored territory by becoming familiar with pertinent issues.

The issues in this chapter are divided into several areas: defining the expanded role; taking on the expanded role; the student role;

professional relationships; professionalism; third party reimbursement; marketing; legal aspects; legislation; and patient-related issues. In reality, many of these areas are intertwined (i.e., taking on the expanded role) and will emerge as crucial issues with some predictability throughout a program. Although most issues are specific to the nurse practitioner role, many will also apply to nurse midwives, nurse anesthetists, and physicians' assistants. The various facets of each issue are briefly explored, but the full development of each is left to the faculty developing new programs. Concepts related to the larger issues are briefly explored. The suggested readings at the end of this chapter can be used as a starting point to research the issues.

DEFINING THE EXPANDED ROLE

What is it? The most complex issue to be faced by students early and often is the basic question "What is a nurse practitioner?" Although the nurse practitioner role was delineated about twenty years ago, controversy and changing views have prevented the development of a universally accepted definition.

From the beginning there was no agreement as to whether the nurse practitioner role was an expanded, extended, or new role in nursing. At one end of the continuum there were nurses who claimed that what the nurse practitioner was doing was not nursing but a physician's assistant role (Rogers, 1972). This controversy might be characterized as the "supernurse versus the junior doctor" discussion. Others who believe that the nurse practitioner role is an expanded role within nursing also believe that many of the current skills and functions will be assumed by baccalaureate- and master's-prepared nurses in the future. This is happening to some extent as many schools are including physical assessment and nursing diagnoses in their programs.

Both intra- and interprofessional conflict have been characterized by the nurse practitioner movement. The question of roles and functions was explored freely within nursing and by early supporters in medicine throughout the 1970s. However, as the supply of physicians grew and a surplus projected in the future (Department of

Health, Education, and Welfare, 1979), opposition to increasing the numbers of nurse practitioners and nurse midwives has grown among physicians.

Throughout the period of role exploration, opposition has also come from within nursing as well. The principal reason given is that the role is outside of nursing. While nursing schools compete for dwindling federal state, and local funds, other specialists in nursing are questioning the need for and the future of a special track or major in primary care. Moreover, there is sometimes little distinction between the nurse practitioner and the clinical specialist. It appears that the roles may be converging to some extent as nurse practitioners move into inpatient settings.

Importance of role issues in the curriculum

The faculty of each program must first decide on their definition of a nurse practitioner. Some guidance is available from nursing organizations and other literature (Bliss & Cohen, 1977; United States Department of Health, Education, and Welfare, 1972) but the operational definition of the particular expanded role must be determined by the faculty. Some components of the definition that should be included are: roles; functions; settings for practice; population served; educational preparation; and professional relationships with other health care disciplines. If funded by external sources, the definition must be agreeable to the funding source.

Once a definition of the expanded role is formulated, the concept is taught as cognitive content and as an affective expectation. That is, students are taught what a nurse practitioner is and are then expected to take on the role.

Role theory

In teaching about conflicting viewpoints of the nurse practitioner role as expanded, extended, or new, it is helpful to structure the discussion in terms of a role theory or theories. Some related concepts are role-taking, role conflict, role strain, role norms, and role prescriptions (Biddle & Thomas, 1966; Hardy & Conway, 1978).

TAKING ON THE EXPANDED ROLE

Nurses are socialized into the traditional nursing role; hence, some authors believe taking on the nurse practitioner or other expanded role is a resocialization process. Malkemes (1974) detailed three phases in the resocialization of nurse practitioner students: unfreezing the role; establishing the role; and role reinforcement. A parallel process described is the move from dependent to interdependent and finally to independent problem solving. She observed a time of role crisis for students in a continuing education program between the first and second phases. Students were confused as to who they were and where they were going. This author has personally experienced this crisis as a student in a continuing education program and observed it repeatedly as a faculty member within a few weeks of the first patient management assignments in a master's program. Early in a program most students are emersed in the technical and medical aspects of the role to the exclusion of their former nursing identity. (This author calls this the "narrow focus" phase.) As the mystique of the physical exam is unveiled and conquered, the nuring role is reintegrated with new roles and functions at varying rates by most students. Parallel to this is an emerging relationship with physicians progressing from dependency to professional intimacy (Anderson, Leonard, & Yates, 1974). Most authors describe a "coming together" later of the care and cure aspects of the expanded role.

Students need to know that their initial confusion and misgivings about the expanded role are typical. Moreover, they can be helped to sort out their feelings and to identify their specific need for help. There are always a few who may, to some degree, not take on a new nursing role but adopt a "junior doctor" role. Others may resist learning new skills and role functions that they believe are not within the purview of nursing. It is helpful to remind the latter that physicians are also expanding into traditional nursing, that is, holistic health care and family, and that some nursing skills, for example, the taking of blood pressures and temperatures, were once done only by physicians. It is not realistic to ignore the gray areas of overlap between medicine and nursing. Each nurse in an expanded role must personally define the boundaries of nursing and related professions while realizing that these boundaries are constantly changing. For example, it may be quite appropriate in an isolated setting for a nurse practitioner to suture wounds and draw blood samples, whereas these tasks should belong to a physician or technician in a large medical center.

THE STUDENT ROLE

At the same time that students are learning a new nursing role, they are taking on another new role, that of student. For some, this may be the more difficult of the two role changes. Most expanded-role programs require some work experience and often seek out nurses who are assertive and exhibit leadership qualities. Students may literally go from a position of great authority and responsibility to a dependent student role where expectations are spelled out in great detail, leaving little decision making to the student. Not only must they be helped to assume the student role, but faculty should examine their attitudes about student behavior. The faculty may know what a student has to learn to become a competent practitioner but there should be an element of colleagueship in the process of teaching adults. Perhaps some of the so-called regressive behavior seen in adult students is precisely because they are being treated and taught as children and consequently living up to the faculty's expectations. Knowledge of principles of adult learning such as respect for diverse opinions should be applied (see Chapter 7) when counseling and teaching professional students.

Nurse practitioners, as other professionals, must prepare for a lifetime of study. The knowledge base in nursing is expanding rapidly so that formal and informal study are necessary to maintain and expand knowledge and skills. Faculty, by role modeling and instilling the value of continuing education, can be instrumental in helping students develop positive attitudes. Faculty should also consider what, if any, responsibility their institution has to provide ongoing education for their graduates.

PROFESSIONAL RELATIONSHIPS

The health care team

A concept related to role is the health care team. Once a nurse decides on a professional role, the relationship with other coworkers must be considered. Who are the members of the team? What are their roles and responsibilities? The nurse practitioner's role on the team varies with setting, patient population, other team members, and most importantly, with the nurse practitioner's conceptualization of the expanded role. Although nurses generally value a team approach, other professionals may not. Role, status, authority, and power are related concepts that can help students understand the dynamics of a health care team and other work groups for that matter. For instance, the physician may be looked upon as an expert in areas not related to medical knowledge because of the relatively greater power of that profession. The idea that the physician may not always be the most effective "captain of the ship" for every patient or population is a good topic for discussion. The student must be made aware of the various relationships—supervision, direction, or collaboration—that are possible between nurse practitioners and physicians.

A concept related to the nurse practitioner role on the health team is that aspect of clinical judgment of knowing one's own limits. A generalist physician must know when to refer to a specialist. Similarly, a nurse in an expanded role must know when to refer to a physician, social worker, or to others more capable of helping the patient. Because of the great variety of backgrounds of nurse practitioners, this decision is difficult to generalize and must be made on a case-by-case basis. A nurse practitioner with experience in coronary intensive care may have depth of knowledge in cardiovascular problems but not in gynecology. A former community health nurse may not need to refer to a social worker as quickly as another practitioner without such experience. The amount of referral depends on expertise, setting, and others on the immediate health care team. Hence, it is important for students to distinguish among collaboration, consultation, and referral.

Comparing and contrasting the role of the nurse practitioner to that of a physician or physician's assistant is a revealing exercise for students when it involves face-to-face discussion. The comparison becomes very complex when the many levels of education preparation that are available for the roles are considered (Bliss & Cohen, 1977).

It is evident that the boundaries of the health professions continue to evolve and perhaps will never be clearly defined. Students need help in dealing with the gray areas of overlap with nursing and other professions. These are not only with medicine, as mentioned earlier, but with other professions such as social work, health education, psychology, and health care administration. Acceptance of ambiguity is a necessary part of taking on an expanded role both in defining the role and in making clinical decisions. Although neophyte professionals want a definitive solution to each clinical and professional relationship problem that develops, faculty can encourage acceptance of several equally cogent alternatives. This includes the ability to avoid jumping to quick conclusions or, conversely, the ability to take a stand when supported by sufficient data. Other useful concepts when studying the health care team are competition, territoriality, negotiation, conflict management, planned change, and the nurse as a change agent.

The health care team and sex roles

An inevitable result of discussion of health team roles is the consideration of sex roles and the health care professions. Most physicians are men; most nurses, and consequently, most nurse practitioners, are women. The issues of power and authority in medicine and nursing are extensions of the same issues in male and female roles. Students and faculty cannot analyze the role of the nurse practitioner or nurse midwife without consideration of the sex role factor (Bullough, 1975). Interdisciplinary groups of students provide an excellent forum for the discussion of these issues early in the educational process. Research studies and other literature are plentiful.

Assertiveness

Assertiveness is a concept receiving much attention in women's professions. Faculty may wish not only to include the concept as content but also provide formal assertiveness training for students and faculty. Observation of assertiveness in various professions in clinical settings is a useful exercise for students. Assertiveness is, to a great extent, inherently necessary in expanded roles because of the need for independent decision making and assurance in working with other professions.

PROFESSIONALISM

A review of the concept of professionalism may be needed, depending on students' previous backgrounds and education. What are the characteristics of a profession? Is nursing a profession? If not, are we moving in that direction? Graduate programs, especially, should examine this issue.

Several professional issues are particularly pertinent to expanded roles. Autonomy is one of these. Mundinger (1980) gives a comprehensive treatment of the subject with an entire chapter devoted to autonomy and the nurse practitioner role.

Accountability

Accountability has become somewhat of an overused buzz word in nursing but it is still important to nurses in expanded roles. In traditional roles, nurses are usually accountable to the institution or to the physician employing them. In primary care settings, accountability shifts, in great measure, to the patient. The ramifications of this change are many. If the nurse practitioner is accountable to the patient and there are disputes on the health care team about patient management, a dilemma occurs. Accountability to the patient adds new meaning to the role that may cause discomfort to students.

Ethical issues

Ethical issues are related to increased accountability and autonomy inherent in the expanded role. Renewed interest in ethics in health care has resulted in considerable literature on the subject. Depending on the patient population served, dilemmas may occur in such areas as family planning, minor consent, the right to die, and quality of life. The increased responsibility for patient management may result in ethical dilemmas in areas such as certification of disability, use of psychotropic drugs, and privileged communication.

Clinical privileges

As nurses who are primary care providers have patients who are admitted to hospitals, they have the choice of turning them over to a physician or of obtaining clinical privileges within hospitals and nursing homes. Unfortunately, most clinical privileges are granted by medical committees. Some hospitals do involve nursing in various ways and plans have been proposed for nursing staff organizations that would grant privileges (Kimbro & Gifford, 1980), but no ideal mechanism is available.

The professional and legal aspects of clinical privileges are important to the development of expanded roles and to independent practice in particular. If committees composed only of physicians grant privileges, are they defining nursing? Should nurses and physicians' assistants take orders from nurse practitioners and nurse midwives? For what functions should privileges be granted? The subject is complex and a matter of great concern for the future in that lack of privileges hampers the practitioner's ability to provide continuity of care.

THIRD PARTY REIMBURSEMENT

Because of the great dependence on health insurance to pay for health care, the extension of third party reimbursement to nurse practitioners is of great urgency. Without reimbursement through insurance, the degree of independence as well as potential income is limited. Students should keep up to date on developments in states where nurses are receiving third party reimbursement.

MARKETING

As students approach the end of their program, they often have misgivings about finding a job or negotiating a new role in their former employment setting. Presenting a class or unit based on the concepts of marketing and packaging is helpful. After a first negative reaction to this approach, most faculty and students find it helpful. The "product" (the nurse prepared for an expanded role) is not known to the potential "buyer" (patients, institutions, physicians) or, if so, the message may be unclear or incorrect. The first step in marketing oneself as a nurse in an expanded role is to decide what you have to sell. Edmunds (1980) suggests that a marketing portfolio is a good selling technique. It includes a resume or curriculum vitae, a position description (Edmunds, 1979), copies of license, certification, malpractice insurance policy, and program completion certificate or transcript. Copies of published and unpublished manuscripts are helpful for positions in teaching or research. Applications for clinical positions are enhanced by patient education or other material developed by the applicant, a list of continuing education programs attended, and references from previous employers and instructors. In Chapter 9, a marketing portfolio is suggested as a student assignment.

Practice sites

In addition to helping students develop the portfolio, faculty can be a clearing house for employment opportunities and act as a coach prior to interviews. Faculty who know the students' strengths and weaknesses can help match the students to first jobs that will promote further development of expertise. Studies show that organizational variables affect the ability of a nurse practitioner to practice (Zammuto, Turner, Miller, Shannon, & Christian, 1979). Students need rudimentary skills in analyzing a health care organization as a possible work site. Some questions to ask are:

- What are the lines of authority?
- Who hires the nurse in the expanded role?
- Who evaluates and how frequently?
- What is the basis for evaluation?
- How is patient care evaluated?
- Who are the members of the health care team?
- What is the degree of collaboration/consultation within the agency?
- What is the apparent level of job satisfaction?
- Are other nurse practitioners or nurse midwives employed?
- Who has the formal and informal power?

Once a student judges an organization to be a potential employer, specific questions related to salary and fringe benefits such as time off for professional development, can be asked in an interview. Wolf (1980) gives specific information on negotiating a contract with a potential employer.

Related to the concept of marketing is the health workforce. Faculty and students should read the GMENAC Report (Department of Health, Education, and Welfare, 1979) and other literature projecting a surplus of physicians later in this century. Does this mean the market for expanded-role nurses will cease to exist? To the contrary, it should motivate nurses to be lucid in interpreting what they have to offer and market it aggressively. The emphasis in a continuing education program should be on marketing the role whereas a graduate program can look at the total health manpower situation in relation to projected needs.

LEGAL ASPECTS OF THE EXPANDED ROLE

Nurse practitioner students and others in expanded roles do not have to be prompted to examine the legal issues inherent in their role. Misinformation and scare tactics can convince students that their newly chosen role is illegal and that they will incur severe penalties.

Practice acts

Legal aspects should be examined on an individual program and state basis because each state will present a different situation. The nurse practice act, the medical practice act, and the pharmacy act together have an impact on practice in an expanded role. Each defines the profession and limits who may practice it. If there is overlap in functions such as the prescription of medicines, both the medical and pharmacy practice acts may define who has the privilege to do so. On the other hand, the nurse practice act itself can limit expanded role functions by narrowly defining nursing. Others may provide for expanded roles, but have additional rules and regulations for the nurse practitioner, nurse midwife, or nurse anesthetist. These rules and regulations list specific roles and functions in greater detail than the nurse practice act. Educational preparation, use of protocols, written agreements with physicians for supervision, and the closeness of that supervision are some of the subjects of specific rules and regulations. For instance, they may specify that the nurse practitioner must be a graduate of an accredited program or that the physician must be within reach by telecommunication at all times.

In some states, joint practice position statements have been made by medical, nursing, and hospital groups. These may offer some protection against being sued for practicing medicine without a license.

Students need to know not only what the legal practice of nursing is in a particular state but also the definitions of related terms such as malpractice, negligence, malfeasance, and liability. It is helpful when studying a state's nurse practice act to delineate the dependent, independent, and interdependent functions of nursing. Students are surprised to find out how much of nursing practice is based on independent decisions and, thus, how much legal responsibility a nurse has even in a traditional role.

Key issues in analyzing a practice act are the inclusion of the ability to diagnose, prescribe, and treat in the definition of nursing. Although some attempts have been made at surveying the status of all state practice acts, the findings are soon outdated (Trandel-Korenchuck & Trandel-Korenchuck, 1980). Up-to-date sources are the individual state boards of nursing, the practice acts, and lawyers who specialize in malpractice and health care litigation. State nurses' associations also offer speakers on legal issues.

Independent and group nursing practice are related topics for student discussion. Increasing numbers are entering expanded role programs to prepare for independent practice. Legal aspects as well as business management are part of the knowledge base needed to pursue independent practice (Koltz, 1979).

Malpractice insurance

After thorough investigation of the legal status of nurses in expanded roles in their state, a discussion of malpractice insurance should follow. The merits of a high liability option should be stressed as well as a thorough examination of the extent of coverage for expanded-role nurses. It is also important to know that malpractice insurance does not protect a nurse against being charged with the practice of medicine. If this is the charge, the insurance company will not defend the nurse under a malpractice policy (Adler, 1979).

Credentialing

Credentialing is a professional issue with legal aspects. As the certification process is becoming more widespread and formalized, states are requiring certification as a condition of practice in expanded roles. Some may give their own examination but most accept the credentials from a national certifying body such as the American Nurses' Association (ANA), the Nurses Association of the American College of Obstetrics and Gynecology (NAACOG), or the National Association of Pediatric Nurse Associates and Practitioners (NAPNAP). Others accept evidence of national certification for certification in the state. Students should be encouraged to pursue certification as a professional responsibility whether or not a particular state requires it. Curriculum content should include the various aspects of professional credentialing including accreditation of programs, licensing, and certification.

LEGISLATION

Legislation is an issue related to legal aspects of practice. Because legislation is the basis for professional acts and has a general impact on health care delivery and financing, students should be alerted to the importance of not only monitoring health-related legislation but of becoming activists in promoting legislation favorable to nursing and to the improvement of health care. As competition in health care delivery increases, recent hard-won gains are being threatened. Vigilence in monitoring a wide variety of legislative topics will be necessary to maintain and gain approval for expanded nursing roles. Some germane topics to oversee are health care financing (including third party reimbursement), licensing of all health care professionals, hospital, nursing home, and home health care regulation, prescriptive authority, and financing of professional education. The legislative committees of all levels of professional organizations are a source of information as various issues emerge in legislative bodies. Students in specialty areas may find it profitable to become active in particular areas such as maternal-child health, alcoholism, safety, abortion rights, adoption or custody, and other human service issues.

The legislative process—state, local, and national—should become familiar to faculty and students. Although time is limited in a continuing education program, the topics should be introduced if only to promote an activist role. In a baccalaureate or master's program more time can be spent on field trips to hearings, visits to legislators' offices, and explaining how political power can be mobilized to influence the legislative process. Lobbying—a new skill for nurses—is the most direct way to influence the legislative process. State nurses' associations and the League of Women Voters are resources for teaching this process. If there are elected public officials who are nurses, they are sources for obtaining information and targets for lobbying for expanded roles.

PATIENT/CLIENT-RELATED ISSUES

Many of the concepts related to patient care are introduced to students in their basic nursing preparation but some may need updating. Even the decision to use the term patient or client is an issue. Some nurses see the use of the term client as indicating a greater mutuality in setting goals. Others use the terms synonymously.

Much literature is now available on patient compliance, an unfortunate term, but of universal use. Students should be aware of their responsibility in facilitating compliance. Techniques in patient education should be reviewed. Some of the behavioral techniques in changing health-related behavior such as biofeedback, self-help groups, and therapeutic touch may be appropriate for inclusion in the curriculum. Counseling techniques for a particular patient group, that is, the elderly, families, or children, add valuable management skills. Most new graduates are amazed at the large psychosomatic and behavioral component in diagnosis and management of problems. Some crisis intervention techniques can be applied in ambulatory as well as acute care settings if developmental tasks of various ages and illness episodes are considered predictable life crises. This viewpoint also prompts the practitioner to involve other resources such as the family or school.

Some concepts speak to the relationship between the patient and the practitioner. Access to patients is a problem for many practitioners. Who controls the nurse's access to patients and how accessible is the nurse to those who prefer nurses as primary care providers? The rise in consumerism in health care is an advantage to the nurse as the public demands alternatives to the traditional health care delivery system. The nurse-patient contract is one approach to involving the patient in his own care.

Of course, the concept of primary care should be introduced early. Developing a personal definition for a particular population and practice site is a useful exercise for students. Aspects of primary care such as health maintenance and disease prevention may not be as familiar to students as illness-orientated topics. The complexity of health screening becomes apparent when a student is asked to develop criteria for screening procedures for various populations. Epidemiology offers a way of approaching health and illness through consideration of risk factors, host, environment, and agent.

SUMMARY

This chapter brings together a wide variety of issues that faculty should consider and include as content when constructing a new program or changing an existing curriculum. Some are issues of interest to all nurses, but they are all of compelling concern to nurses in expanded roles. Nearly all could be classified as relationship issues—either with patients, other nurses, other disciplines, or future employers. Although exploration of the concepts identified help prepare students for the difficult and unpredictable professional future, others are likely to surface. Faculty should be prepared to deal with them on a personal level and then integrate them into the curriculum.

REFERENCES

Adler, J. 'You are charged with . . .' *Nurse Practitioner*, 1979, *4*, (1), 45–46.

American Nurses' Association, Division on Community Health Nursing Practice. *Guidelines for short-term continuing education programs preparing adult and family nurse practitioners.* Kansas City: American Nurses' Association, 1975.

Anderson, E. M., Leonard, B. J. & Yates, J. A. Epigenesis of the nurse practitioner role. *American Journal of Nursing*, 1974, *74*, 1812–1816.

Biddle, B. J. & Thomas, E. J. (Eds.). *Role theory: Concepts and research.* New York: John Wiley and Sons, 1966.

Bliss, A. A. & Cohen, E. D. (Eds.). *The new health professionals: Nurse practitioners and physician's assistants.* Germantown, Maryland: Aspen Systems Corporation, 1977.

Bullough, B. Barriers to the nurse practitioner movement: Problems of women in a woman's field. *International Journal of Health Services*, 1975, *5*, 225–233.

Department of Health, Education, and Welfare (HEW), Public Health Service, Health Resources Administration, Office of Graduate Medical Education. Interim report of the graduate medical education national advisory committee (GMENAC). Hyattsville, Maryland: Department of Health, Education, and Welfare, 1979.

Edmunds, M. The position description. *Nurse Practitioner*, 1979, *4* (4), 45–47.

Edmunds, M. Developing a marketing portfolio. *Nurse Practitioner*, 1980, *5* (5), 41, 43, 46.

Ford, L. & Silver, H. K. The expanded role of the nurse in child care. *Nursing Outlook*, 1967, *15*, 43–45.

Hardy, M. E. & Conway, M. E. *Role theory: Perspectives for health professionals.* New York: Appleton-Century-Crofts, 1978.

Kimbro, C. D. & Gifford, A. J. The nursing staff organization: A needed development. *Nursing Outlook*, 1980, *28* (10), 610–616.

Koltz, C. J. *Private practice in nursing: Development and management.* Germantown, Maryland: Aspen Systems Corporation, 1979.

Malkemes, L. C. Resocialization: A model for nurse practitioner preparation. *Nursing Outlook*, 1974, *22*, 90–94.

Mundinger, M. O. *Autonomy in nursing.* Germantown, Maryland: Aspen Systems Corporation, 1980.

Rogers, M. Nursing: To be or not to be. *Nursing Outlook*, 1972, *20*, 42–46.

Trandel-Korenchuck, D. M. & Trandel-Korenchuck, K. M. Current legal issues facing nursing practice. *Nursing Administration Quarterly*, 1980, *5* (1), 37–45.

United States Department of Health, Education, and Welfare. Committee to Study Extended Roles for Nurses. Extending the scope of nursing practice. *Nursing Outlook*, 1972, *20*, 46–52.

Wolf, G. A. Negotiating an employment contract. *Nurse Practitioner*, 1980, *5* (1), 55, 60.

Zammuto, R. F., Turner, I. R., Miller, S., Shannon, I. & Christian, J. Effect of clinical settings on the utilization of nurse practitioners. *Nursing Research*, 1979, *28* (2), 98–102.

SUGGESTED READINGS

Bakker, C. B. & Bakker-Rabdau, M. K. *No trespassing! Explorations in human territoriality.* San Francisco: Chandler and Sharp Publishers, Inc., 1973.

Balassone, P. D. Territorial issues in an interdisciplinary experience. *Nursing Outlook*, 1981, *29*, 229–232.

Bliss, A. A. & Cohen, E. D. Issues confronting the new health professions. *Journal of Allied Health*, 1978, *7*, 64–72.

Committee for the Study of Credentialing in Nursing. Credentialing in nursing: A new approach. *American Journal of Nursing*, 1979, *79*, 674–683.

Duncanis, A. J. & Golin, A. K. *The interdisciplinary health care team.* Germantown, Maryland: Aspen Systems Corporation, 1979.

Edmunds, M. Conflict. *Nurse Practitioner*, 1979, *4* (6), 42, 47–48.

Fox, J. G. & Zatkin, S. R. Third party payment for non-physician health practitioners: Realities and recommendations. *Family and Community Health*, 1978, *1* (1), 69–80.

Garfield, S. R. The delivery of primary care. *Scientific American*, 1970, *222* (4), 15–23.

Goldwater, M. From a legislator: Views on third party reimbursement for nurses. *American Journal of Nursing*, 1982, *82*, 411–414.

Griffith, H. M. Strategies for direct third-party reimbursement for nurses. *American Journal of Nursing*, 1982, *82*, 408–411.

Jacox, A. K. & Norris, C. M. (Eds.). *Organizing for independent nursing practice.* New York: Appleton-Century-Crofts, 1977.

Leitch, J. C. & Mitchell, E. S. A state-by-state report: The legal accommodation of nurses practicing in expanded roles. *Nurse Practitioner*, 1977, *2*, (8), 19–22, 30.

Parker, A. W. The dimensions of primary care: Blueprint for change. In Andreopoulis, S. (Ed.), *Primary care: Where medicine fails.* New York: John Wiley and Sons, 1974.

Schachtel, B. P. The pediatric nurse practitioner: Origins and challenges. *Medical Care*, 1978, *16*, 1019–1026.

Scheffler, R. M., Yoder, S. G., Weisfeld, N., & Ruby, G. Physician and new health practitioners: Issues for the 1980s. *Inquiry*, *16*, 195–229.

Weston, J. L. Distribution of nurse practitioners and physicians' assistants: Implications of legal constraints and reimbursement. *Public Health Reports*, 1980, *95*, 253–258.

II

Program Development

3

Preparation of Faculty

Thomasine D. Guberski

The evolution of the nurse practitioner as a primary care provider has had an impact on the development and implementation of faculty roles by those nurse faculty engaged in the education of nurse practitioners. The main difference between the role of the nurse faculty preceptor in primary care and that of other nursing faculty is the assumption of responsibility and accountability for independently and collaboratively providing primary care services to patients. Ongoing, continuous practice as a primary care provider is an integral part of the role for primary care faculty. The nursing faculty teaching primary care blend the responsibilities of college or university faculty member with those of a primary care health provider. The major educational function of the nurse faculty preceptor is to facilitate the development of the student as a primary health care provider. The unique contribution of the nursing faculty is to help the student integrate the new skills of assessment and management into an expanded and evolving nursing role.

Faculty teaching primary care are currently prepared in three ways. Experienced faculty with master's degrees in other specialties often obtain their primary care skills and knowledge in a continuing education certificate program. Some faculty are prepared at the master's level for the dual role of nurse practitioner-educator. Others first complete a certificate program to prepare primary care nurse practitioners, then complete a master's program in primary care or another specialty. A small number of faculty are prepared in primary care doctoral programs.

Regardless of the avenue of entry selected, all nurse faculty should have formal preparation in educational theory and primary care. Formal preparation in education provides a theoretical base on which the prospective faculty member can build her own teaching style. Ideally, the educational foundation would include graduate courses in nursing theory and practice, human cognition and learning, curriculum theory and development, and teaching methodologies. A teaching practicum provides the opportunity for a prospective teacher to practice the behaviors inherent in the faculty role, experience a variety of realistic teaching-learning situations, and test out different teaching methodologies.

The curriculum to prepare nurse practitioners is described in detail in Chapter 6 of this book. This chapter will focus on factors in the development of the nurse faculty preceptor role and on factors affecting the implementation of the role such as continued clinical practice, continuing education, and organizational constraints.

ROLE DEVELOPMENT

In nursing, faculty teaching primary care must be committed to nursing, as well as being competent educators and competent primary care providers. The development of the faculty role is related to the educational program selected for entry since the different types of programs prepare nurse practitioners for different roles and levels of practice. The development and implementation of the faculty role in primary care is a resocialization process. The faculty member must function successfully in a multitask role combining practice, education, research, and consultation. Since few primary care faculty are prepared at the doctoral level, many are enrolled in doctoral programs. Multiple tasks lead to conflicting expectations which must be integrated into one role that fits the faculty member and the institution well. It is imperative that the end result of the resocialization be a nurse practitioner-faculty member qualified to serve as a role model for students and other faculty.

Faculty selected to teach in the nurse practitioner program must be assertive in communicating their functioning and purpose to physician and nurse colleagues. The implementation of a relatively new role requires flexibility to try out different methods of meeting personal, professional, and institutional needs. The person needs to have appropriate coping behaviors because of the uncertainty surrounding the role and the differing expectations of other faculty. The faculty member should be a skilled provider with a strong base in nursing and primary care and have demonstrated the ability to function interdependently with other health care professionals. These characteristics are helpful to new primary care faculty as they modify their former role to integrate the knowledge and skills of a health care provider and educator.

In addition to role changes, primary care faculty must reassure other faculty in the institution of their credibility and accountability as both a faculty member and a nurse practitioner. Having academic credentials is very important in a system where the doctorate usually is considered the minimum degree for appointment, promotion, and/or tenure because many primary care faculty are not doctorally prepared. The doctorate also increases the possibility of being on committees and in influential positions where support for the nurse practitioner curriculum can be built.

In modifying roles, the experienced educator with a post-master's certificate in primary care must cope with integrating primary care skills and knowledge into a well-established faculty role concept while gaining confidence and competence as a primary care provider, frequently while teaching primary care to others. Practitioners who become faculty after being clinical providers of care have been well socialized into the practitioner role but must cope with integrating faculty responsibilities with the familiar role of provider while teaching their skills as a provider to others in formally structured teaching-learning situations.

Role development consists of three phases, role identification, role implementation, and role verification. Role identification consists of clarifying the purposes and objectives of the role both for oneself and for others (Oda, 1977). This is generally accomplished in formal programs where theories of primary care practice and education are presented and discussed. In clinical practice associated with clinical primary care courses, opportunities to implement the nurse practitioner role are provided. If nursing faculty teach in these courses, the opportunity to observe others implementing the role is available. Teaching practicums allow the potential faculty member to practice some of the behaviors inherent in the teaching role. These structured learning situations provide verification of the role; however, they do not provide the opportunity to experience all the expectations inherent in the role of a nurse faculty preceptor. The purposes and objectives of the role can be identified in the abstract, but only experience as a preceptor will result in the integration of all the necessary skills.

The practical purposes and functions of the role are identified when the faculty member is appointed to a specific academic rank in a particular institution. Role identification in a specific organization becomes a mutual interactive process between the individual, peers, subordinates, and superordinates. General responsibilities for teaching, research, and community service for each academic rank are contained in the job description for each rank. Specific responsibilities for research, student contact hours, course responsibilities, clinical precepting, student advisement, committee responsibilities, and other organizational maintenance functions are usually negotiated within the department or similar organizational structural unit. These parameters help clarify the role, yet maintain flexibility for individual role identification.

Role identification

In the role identification phase, communication between the individual and other faculty serves to mutually clarify purposes and beliefs about the role. In addition, philosophical beliefs about nursing practice and primary care can be delineated and areas of agreement and disagreement identified.

Seasoned nurse faculty preceptors have commented that teaching health assessment skills to beginning nurse practitioner students seems to be the least stressful introduction to the precepting role (Helmuth & Guberski, 1980). When an experienced nurse faculty preceptor is paired with a novice, the first teaching experience in primary care is similar to an individually designed advanced teaching practicum. The pairing method provides the less experienced faculty the opportunity to discuss all aspects of the faculty role with a peer. Exposure to more experienced faculty aids in role identification, builds confidence and collegial relationships, and provides opportunities for collaboration. In addition, the success or failure of the use of different teaching methods in teaching primary care can be learned from colleagues rather than from trial and error (Hamilton, 1981).

The experienced educator with limited clinical experience in primary care is likely to need assistance in identifying the clinical precepting responsibilities in the faculty role. Consequently, the experienced clinician with limited teaching experience is likely to need assistance in the teaching, research, and service aspects of the role. The novice teacher needs help in identifying methods of student advisement, realistic work loads in regard to didactic teaching and committee work, and her need for development as a faculty member. Exploring the epigenesis of the faculty role with peers and colleagues is frequently beneficial in clarifying role expectations and identifying potential conflict areas before they become a problem.

Role implementation: the preceptor

The implementation of the nurse preceptor role will vary from program to program and from institution to institution. The common elements in role implementation will be discussed in this section.

The most critical aspect of implementing the nurse faculty preceptor role is to provide support for the student as she develops her own concept and skills as a primary care nurse practitioner. The relationship between faculty and students tends to evolve from a student-teacher relationship early in the educational program to a more collegial relationship later in the educational program. The teaching of advanced nurse practitioner students is facilitated by an increased level of confidence in one's ability as a provider and educator. Clinical precepting situations in which the faculty assumes varying degrees of responsibility for the clinical diagnosis and management of patients is frequently a source of stress for the less experienced nurse preceptor. The role of copreceptor with a physician or another nurse faculty member reduces the stress and builds sophistication in the precepting process. As faculty become more comfortable with the level of uncertainty that exists in the clinical situation, they are able to utilize the physician more in a consultative/collaborative role than as the primary care decision maker. As the nurse faculty preceptor gains confidence in her role, she is more able to encourage students to assume increased responsibility for patient care in appropriate situations.

An integral part of developing the nurse faculty preceptor role is the establishment of a collegial relationship with the consulting physician preceptors. Nourishing a collegial relationship requires that each person has a secure professional role identity. This provides the professional background for the confidence and trust which comes with joint practice.

The establishment of a collegial relationship with the physician preceptor is also a process of mutual role development. Initially the dependent decision-making role assumed by the neophyte nurse faculty preceptor is comfortable for both the nurse and the physician preceptor. The physician assumes the role of teacher and primary decision maker, and the nurse faculty is the student. The assessment of psychosocial health problems, areas in which the nurse faculty excels, tends to be temporarily ignored while the nurse concentrates on the physical diagnosis and management of physiological problems. The emphasis on physical diagnosis and management by the physician combined with uncertainty about the role of the nurse faculty often produces a crisis for the nurse, with the individual asking "How should I function in this situation?"

As the nurse faculty preceptor gains confidence in her decision-making ability, her need for physician support and guidance diminishes and the nurse focuses on independent decision making. This is often difficult for the physician to accept. Some physicians perceive a loss of control of the clinical situation, especially if they do not have confidence in the nurse's decision-making ability. During this stage the nurse faculty preceptor often feels as if she must prove herself and her ability to the physician, while teaching students to become primary care providers. Meanwhile the nurse is unconsciously or consciously evaluating the physician as a preceptor. A positive resolution of the conflict that often arises during this stage leads to increased knowledge of the role of the nurse faculty preceptor by the physician and a collegial relationship (Malkemes, 1974).

The transition to a collegial precepting relationship occurs when both nurse faculty and physician preceptor feel confident in what each uniquely brings to the precepting situation and trust in each other's decision-making abilities. Generally the physician brings an in-depth knowledge of diagnostic and treatment modalities for less common and acute health problems, and greater depth of knowledge of the pathophysiology of disease. Nursing faculty generally have a broader knowledge base in health maintenance and the assessment and management of psychosocial problems.

Crisis points in the epigenesis of the nurse practitioner role have been identified (Anderson, Leonard, & Yates, 1974). The most frequent is the temporary loss of a nursing focus. As a nurse practitioner with a strong and well-articulated nursing identity, the nurse faculty facilitates the student's socialization by assisting the students to integrate their previous identity with nursing into their role as a primary care provider of health care. In each learning experience it is the responsibility of the nursing faculty to foster the student's utilization of previous nursing knowledge and use of theories for nursing practice in addition to primary care concepts and skills. This is one way to integrate the "nurse" into the role of nurse practitioner.

In the educational program, the nursing faculty have primary responsibility for structuring the student's learning experiences. The experiences should be structured to provide the students with the knowledge and skills necessary to: (1) assess the whole person, including his strengths and deficits, by gathering pertinent data, (2) organize the data in a logical, concise manner using a problem-solving approach, (3) identify the health needs/patient problems including potential problems, (4) devise a rational, individualized plan of management with the patient, including nursing goals and follow-up, (5) provide patient education that will enhance self-care abilities, (6) be a patient advocate, and (7) demonstrate accountability as a primary care provider.

The student's clinical experiences should be designed to allow the student to apply the information from the classroom to specific patient situations. The student should be viewed as the primary provider with the faculty assuming varying levels of responsibility for data gathering and validation of data, for problem identification and management, and for patient education. The student should be able to identify her own realistic strengths and limitations as a primary care provider. The level of responsibility for patient care assumed by the faculty depends on the ability of the student, the complexity of the patient's health problems, and the confidence of the faculty member in her own decision-making ability.

In the clinical setting, the nurse faculty preceptor frequently has the opportunity to be a role model for the student interested in teaching as a future career. Interaction with patients to validate critical aspects of the data base gives the faculty member an opportunity to demonstrate additional interviewing and assessment techniques to the student. When the faculty member critiques the student's formal presentation of the student-patient interaction, the other students have additional opportunities to learn the "art" of managing various health problems.

Role verification

Role verification is provided by student, peers, and superordinates. Most role verification is provided in a mentor relationship. Although mentoring has not been used as much in nursing as in predominantly male professions (Hamilton, 1981), aspects have been used in developing faculty in primary care. The functions of a mentor are to provide guidance, support, and consultation, and to act as a role model to the less experienced colleague. Relevant information shared in the mentor relationship includes orientation to the political system of the institution, including the formal policies and procedures and the norms of the informal system. Role verification is also facilitated by providing guidance for the neophyte in setting and meeting professional goals. The more experienced faculty can offer praise and constructive criticism about role implementation and offer specific suggestions for improvement. This type of interaction with other faculty reinforces role definition.

The three stages of role development are not mutually exclusive. Role development is a continuous process for the faculty member in primary care since the role of the nurse practitioner is constantly evolving. In the current time of decreasing enrollments and financial constraints, faculty are being forced to reevaluate their roles and functioning.

ROLE IMPLEMENTATION

Clinical practice

Continued clinical practice as a provider is vital to maintain and improve skills as a nurse faculty preceptor. Clinical practice must meet the needs of the individual and the institution.

Clinical practice in an interdisciplinary health care team is the means by which nurse faculty preceptors are exposed to a variety of health care professionals and their unique approaches to dealing with patient problems. It is also a means of continuing credibility with students and reinforces the view of faculty as a role model. Continued contact with clinicians helps keep faculty abreast of clinical issues and builds and strengthens collegial relationships. Active involvement in patient care is the best method available to maintain and improve skills as a primary care provider.

Practice privileges should be negotiated as part of faculty responsibilities. In negotiating with a specific site, the positive aspects of having a faculty nurse practitioner associated with the practice should be stressed. Faculty can provide in-service for other nurse practitioners or nurses in the practice site. Since faculty are also experts in nursing care, they are valuable resources in establishing standards of practice for nursing care and in establishing and/or conducting peer audits. In addition, nurse practitioners are well accepted by patients as providers of care and they increase profits in most practice settings.

The question of reimbursement for clinical practice should be decided early in the process of negotiating with a clinical practice site. Reimbursement in some form should be actively pursued prior to beginning practice since people rarely value free service. Reimbursement can be a salary paid to the faculty member, a fee for service arrangement with the individual, payment to the educational institution, or an agreement that the clinical site will provide educational experiences and/or preceptors for students in exchange for faculty clinical practice. A joint appointment between the school of nursing and the clinical facility helps to legitimize the responsibilities for both practice and teaching.

The greatest source of conflict for most nurse practitioner faculty seems to be juggling patient care with education and/or research. Ongoing clinical practice is a weekly commitment for most nurse practitioner faculty. This limits the flexibility of scheduling other activities since clinical commitments are difficult to change. Other faculty and nursing school administration frequently view clinical practice as an add-on to other faculty responsibilities. In some practice settings the faculty member is seen as a "dabbler" because of a limited time commitment to practice. Other providers in the practice setting may also resent the limited time faculty are able to practice because they must see the faculty member's patients when the faculty member is not available. Arrangements for providing back-up personnel to see patients when the faculty member is not available should be made with the clinical practice site during the negotiation process. Expectations should be clarified and a mutual understanding of the rights and responsibilities of both parties should be reached.

Since health care professionals tend to identify with the profession and its values first and with the organization and its goals second, many nurse practitioner faculty feel guilty over the conflicts caused by patient care. A partial answer to the conflict is to negotiate roles and responsibilities carefully in each organization. In the school of nursing, clinical practice for primary care faculty must be viewed as an integral part of the role. The academic reward system needs to give faculty credit for clinical practice just as consultation or serving on professional committees is rewarded. If the school of nursing is part of an academic medical center with other health professional schools, policies governing faculty practice and its place in the reward system may have been established by other schools. If these policies exist, they can be adapted to meet the needs of the nursing faculty.

Continuing education

Nursing faculty engaged in teaching primary care should be certified by their professional association. Requirements for continuing education are specified in the recertification requirements of the American Nurses' Association and for relicensure in some states. Continuing education should be in the field of education and primary care. Continuing education in primary care can be obtained in a variety of settings. Medical grand rounds is one source of continuing education which provides the faculty with clinically current information. Peer audits are another form of continuing education. Peer audits provide the faculty with the opportunity to measure their standards of care against standards held by other experts in the field. Short courses or formal credit-awarding courses in nursing or medicine will help faculty keep current or extend their knowledge.

Pharmacology is another area for continuing education. These sessions should be conducted by clinical pharmacists and geared toward the rational use of therapeutics in the treatment of patient health problems.

Attending national or regional meetings for nurse practitioners provides nursing faculty the opportunity to learn new developments in their field and to interact with faculty from other institutions to discuss techniques of teaching primary care.

For those faculty who have minimal preparation in curriculum and instruction, continuing education and credit courses in topics such as test construction, nursing theory, measurement, and educational administration are possibilities.

Organizational constraints

The organizational structure exerts a strong influence on the implementation of the nurse faculty preceptor role. Traditionally, industrial organizational models have been used as the basis for organizing academic institutions. In the industrial model, each member of the organization has one task and is accountable to one person for task performance. In academe, however, each faculty member is expected to contribute to the attainment of the institution's three goals:

teaching, research, and community service. This leads to potential conflict between tasks. Faculty are accountable to the department chairman for all tasks. Nurse faculty preceptors must meet the same expectations and responsibilities as other faculty. In addition, they must integrate their clinical practice with their other faculty responsibilities. In reality, a different system of accountability exists, although in many institutions it is informal. The department chairman is the administrator to whom each faculty is accountable for all matters regarding education and time spent in other university settings. When the faculty member is involved in doing research, the faculty is accountable to the project director. The physician and/or nurse administrator in the clinical setting hold the faculty accountable as a provider in their setting. Therefore, the individual nurse faculty preceptor is inherently placed in conflict in each area of responsibility. Both the organizational structure and the informal structure require an individual to perform several diverse tasks within the faculty role.

SUMMARY

Since primary care is a rather new specialty, it is often misunderstood, frequently by other nurses. One major task in the development and implementation of the faculty role in primary care is explaining the role to other faculty. The role is unique in nursing and combines the role of primary health care provider and educator. The development of the role is a three-phased interactive and cyclical process. Developing and maintaining high-level functioning as a nurse faculty preceptor is a demanding task that requires continued practice as a primary care provider and continuing education while fulfilling teaching and other professional responsibilities.

REFERENCES

Anderson, E. M., Leonard, B. J., & Yates, J. A. Epigenesis of the nurse practitioner role. *American Journal of Nursing*, 1974, 74 (10), 1812–1816.
Hamilton, M. S. Mentorhood: A key to nursing leadership. *Nursing Leadership*, 1981, 4 (1), 4–13.

Helmuth, M. R. & Guberski, T. D. Preparation for preceptor role. *Nursing Outlook*, 1980, *28*, (1), 36–39.

Malkemes, L. C. Resocialization: A model for nurse practitioner preparation. *Nursing Outlook*, 1974, *22*, (2), 90–94.

Oda, D. Specialized role development: A three-phase process. *Nursing Outlook*, 1977, *25*, (6), 374–377.

4

Student Admissions

Of the many dilemmas in professional education, the selection of students for admission remains one of the most difficult. The problem of choosing students for nurse practitioner graduate, undergraduate, or short courses is that of all professional educators. Some of the perennial questions are:

1. Should only those who are most assured of completing the program be admitted?
2. How do you predict success?
3. Should professionals be selected from groups who need their services most?
4. Should those who can pay their own way be admitted before those needing financial aid?
5. In a state institution, how many out-of-state students should be admitted?
6. Should any effort be made to "balance" programs within a school or department?
7. Which needs should be considered first in determining composition and size of a program—that of society, the school, the profession, or the individual?

Although the questions may be more specific when considering individual applications, these are some of the larger policy questions that faculty face.

IMPORTANCE OF ADMISSION CRITERIA

Because access to education has such a profound formative effect on those who influence society (in this case, the health care delivery system), the admission process is a major link between the social responsibility of higher education and its educational goals. Professional specialty training, whether in short continuing education courses or in degree-granting programs, is a powerful vehicle for upward mobility. This is particularly true in nursing, a profession made up of women predominantly who are seeking meaningful and well-paid employment. The independence of the nurse practitioner role attracts many nurses who (1) hope for more control of their practice; (2) want to exert more leadership in their profession; or, (3) want more professional respect and recognition.

RECENT TRENDS IN ADMISSIONS

Policies and trends in college admissions have usually mirrored societal concerns. Consequently, two major divergent viewpoints on admissions developed in the 1960s. The meritocratic concept held that access to higher education should be solely determined by academic talent without regard to social or economic factors. The opposing egalitarian position declared just as firmly that the methods for determining academic talent are inherently discriminatory for those of certain social and economic backgrounds. The two viewpoints still have strong advocates in most colleges and universities although public institutions tend to be more egalitarian and the private ones more meritocratic in their selection process (Shulman, 1977).

Even more recently other forces have influenced the admissions process. Numerous court decisions including the Bakke decision (1978) and Title IX of the Education Amendments of 1972 barring sex discrimination have made admissions decisions even more complex and subject to litigation. Furthermore, the decrease in numbers of potential students is another factor. As the birth rate falls, the postwar "bulge" in the school population will have completed college and fewer students will be entering higher education programs. A third factor peculiar to nursing and other traditionally female professions is the wider choice of professions women now have. To some, nursing has a negative, subservient image. On the other hand, the nurse practitioner role attracts others who might leave nursing for other fields. For several reasons, the outlook for admissions to nursing programs is changing in the 1980s. While schools may want to attract and admit students with defined characteristics, the potential pool is decreasing.

SELECTING ADMISSIONS CRITERIA

The previous section points out the importance of examining where a college, school, department, and faculty stand on the meritocratic-egalitarian continuum. Potential admissions criteria must reflect this stance while being realistic about the potential applicant pool. In addition, the admissions process must meet minimal legal procedural requirements: "Uniformity of application and fair administration of the regulations" (Gellhorn & Hornby, 1974, p. 997). In other words, although admissions criteria may reflect the goals of the program or school, they must be ascertainable, disseminated to applicants, and applied uniformly and impartially.

One medical school legally chose applicants to a special program to train primary care physicians using personal criteria that selected those most likely to practice in a rural primary care site (Elliott, 1975). Hence, selected personal, personality, or demographic characteristics as well as academic credentials can be used as admission criteria as long as they are made known, fairly administered, and uniformly applied to all applicants. Moreover, the requirements published in school bulletins may be construed as a contract, that is, the school can be held to the admissions information in their catalogs (Rethwisch & Fowler, 1980).

ACADEMIC CRITERIA

Grade-point average (GPA)

The most commonly accepted criteria are those that purport to determine academic achievement or potential to achieve. GPA in high school or previous college work has long been known to be a good predictor of later grades in college. The caution in a nurse practitioner program is to realize that a high GPA may indicate an ability to play the academic game but may not be an indicator of true scholastic ability or the ability to learn new psychomotor skills and combine them to problem-solve in the diagnostic process. Other precautions with the use of GPA are consideration of the expectations or reputation of the school awarding the grades and the number of years the student has been out of school. Mature, competent adults may have a poor record in early college years or in their basic nursing program for many reasons, yet have progressed professionally and have potential for completing further education successfully.

Still, GPA is a valid admissions criterion if used judiciously. Trends upward or downward and grades for particular courses (biological sciences, nursing, behavioral sciences) can indicate a student's strengths and weaknesses. Trends upward in later courses may indicate increasing motivation if the courses are of equal difficulty and applicable to nurse practitioner education.

Writing skills

Nursing requires skills in written communication whether in record keeping or with colleagues and patients. The ability to write cogently and coherently is a skill necessary for academic success. An essay or statement of goals can be used to assess the level of writing ability. Writing on "Why I want to be a nurse practitioner" can demonstrate the ability to organize, write, and spell as well as reveal knowledge of the role. In addition, a writing sample can be used as a diagnostic test to predict the need for remedial instruction.

Standardized tests

College admissions test scores have long been used by the more competitive schools as a screening device. As colleges were glutted with a large number of students in the 1960s and 1970s, the "numbers game" became very important. Similar tests are required for admission to graduate and professional schools. Most are administered by the Educational Testing Service (ETS). Recently, ETS and standardized tests generally have come under fire. There is little doubt that most such tests are culturally biased toward white, middle- and upper-class, native-born Americans. In fact, Scholastic Aptitude Tests scores (SAT) correlate directly with income level. Once touted as a test of intelligence, it is now admitted that the SAT and the companion Graduate Record Examination (GRE) are tests of developed ability. Students who have a good scholastic background learn the test-taking skills, vocabulary, math, and reading skills that increase scores on the standardized test. Minority students' average scores are below those of the total population on ETS-administered tests and many other standardized tests.

To compound the difficulties of interpreting standardized tests, it is now well substantiated that coaching can raise standardized test scores a great deal (Levy, 1979). Formal and expensive prep courses are available to prepare for the GRE as well as the SAT and other professional admissions tests. As an aside, ETS also administers the national nurse practitioner certification examination for the American Nurses' Association. So it is possible that admission to and successful completion of advanced professional education may be influenced by the same group of test makers.

Should standardized testing as an admission criterion be abandoned? Some believe so. At the least, any one score should not be used as a cut-off point for admissions. Typically GPA and SAT or ACT (American College Test) are used as academic indicators for undergraduate admissions while GRE and GPA are used for graduate nursing programs. The Miller Analogy Test is also commonly used and is primarily a vocabulary analogy test.

NONACADEMIC CRITERIA

Work experience

If admission to a postgraduate short course or to a graduate program for nurse practitioners is the reader's concern, a work requirement should be considered. Many teachers of nurse practitioners believe that identity and skills as a nurse must be firm before taking on an expanded role. The amount and character of such experience should be predetermined. One to two years is the usual requirement and should assure competence in nursing in one patient population or specialty area. Some possible areas to examine are:

- experience is relevant and recent
- experience is in both inpatient and outpatient settings
- evidence of professional growth
- evidence of career planning
- evidence of progressive responsibility and leadership

The interpretation of these criteria will vary with the type of nurse practitioner program. For instance, an obstetrics-gynecology (Ob-gyn) program may want to require some inpatient obstetrical experience. Prospective students who seem to be changing specialty areas or patient age groups should be evaluated for their motivation and probability of success in a new area. A student with only experience in adult nursing who wishes to become a pediatric nurse practitioner may well not have the required baseline skills and knowledge to succeed in an expanded role.

Professional activity

Prospective students who have taken the initiative to attend continuing education offerings, be active in professional and community organizations, and read professional journals should be ranked higher than those who have not. Professional and academic honors and awards should also be noted.

Personal characteristics

The practice of choosing students who have certain personal characteristics is controversial. Several studies have assessed the psychological characteristics of nurse practitioners. Baccalaureate nursing students were found to score high in nurturance, deference, order, abasement, and endurance on the Edward's Personal Preference Schedule. Entering nurse practitioner students in the same school scored lower on these traits but higher on autonomy, exhibition, dominance, change, and heterosexuality. Moreover, nurse practitioner students were above average on the self-actualization section of the Personal Orientation Inventory while the baccalaureate students were below the mean (White, 1975).

Certainly the nurse practitioner role requires more autonomy, accountability, and assertiveness than the more traditional nursing role, but choosing students on predetermined characteristics may be risky. Undoubtedly, there is more than one combination of traits that is predictive of success. More complex research is necessary before personality traits can be used as definitive admission criteria.

Other characteristics such as age and maturity may be considered. Ability to withstand academic stress and the presence of support systems may help in surviving the rigors of a graduate or intensive continuing education program.

Motivation and interest are indicated in part by prospective students having talked with and observed the practice of other nurse practitioners and their being able to discuss the role and functions with some accuracy and depth. Self-awareness is a valuable asset in any role change and can be indicated by the ability to write or verbalize one's strengths and weaknesses. Commitment to the new role may be judged by realistic plans to meet the demands of the program and the formalization of future career goals.

PRECEPTOR SUPPORT

In some continuing education courses the student comes from a specific work setting and returns in a new role. If this is the case, the commitment of the physician preceptor and other nurses to facilitate the student's continued learning and to the interprofessional delivery of health care must be assessed. The preceptor must have a clear concept as to the needs, capabilities, and limitations of a nurse who has just completed a nurse practitioner course. The patient population and facilities should be adequate for expanded practice. If there is the customary preceptorship following the didactic portion, there must be mutual planning for proper supervision on the student's return. A site visit is the best way to assess all these factors.

SOURCES OF DATA

Academic transcripts indicate the GPA and grades in salient subjects. The student is urged to submit all records of courses taken beyond the basic nursing preparation whether used for a degree or not. Faculty may wish to weight recent grades more than those earned five or more years ago. Standardized test scores should be forwarded by the testing agency.

Recommendations from peers, superiors, and former instructors form the basis for judging quality of work experience, nursing skills, leadership and organizational ability, personality characteristics, and the ability to cope with stress. Opinions of the references should be consonant with the student's self-evaluation. The number and source of references should be standardized to assure a variety of input. Similarly, the format of the questions should be thoughtfully prepared so that the necessary information is obtained. A checklist does not give as much information as a narrative format.

Interviews

Interviewing prospective students is time-consuming, but the information gained makes the effort worthwhile. Particularly in a program that prepares for an expanded or new role, the interviewer can probe knowledge, attitudes, commitment, and resources in a way impossible with only written records. Also, the prospective student can elaborate on the written data as well as ask questions about the program. In fact, the interview should become a two-way exchange. If necessary, interviews can be conducted by long-distance telephone but are more productive in person.

A scoring system can be used based on the predetermined admissions criteria. This is completed by those responsible for reviewing the records and interviewing. Thus, a somewhat objective method of selecting students can be developed. For instance, a range of scores pertaining to professional activities might include:

	1	2	3	4
a)	No C.E. since graduation	Attends C.E. in own agency	Multiple C.E. in several areas	Plans and/or teaches C.E. offering
b)	No professional organization memberships	Belongs to state ANA— does not attend meetings	Serves on local or state committees	Serves as officer in professional organization
c)	Not able to cite recent professional readings	Subscribes to professional journals	Can discuss journal articles related to NP role	Able to verbalize how reading is integrated into practice

After a number of students has completed the program, it is possible to analyze the predictive validity of total and partial scores on such an instrument.

SUMMARY

Criteria for admission to nurse practitioner programs should reflect the direction and purpose of the parent institution and of the program itself. Criteria can be developed for academic records and background characteristics, scores on standardized or teacher-made tests, work experience, and personal and professional characteristics. Criteria must be well disseminated and applied fairly and uniformly to all prospective students to avoid litigation.

Sources of data for admissions decisions are transcripts, test scores, references, and personal interviews. A scoring method based on predetermined criteria facilitates selection if there are more qualified applicants than can be admitted.

REFERENCES

Elliott, P. R. The selection of primary care physicians. Paper presented at the Workshop for Undergraduate Educators in Family Medicine. American Academy of Family Physicians, Kansas City, Missouri, May 12–14, 1975.

Federal Register, Nondiscrimination on the basis of sex. June 4, 1975, pp. 24128–24144.

Gellhorn, E. & Hornby, D. B. Constitutional limitations on admissions procedures and standards: Beyond affirmative action. *Virginia Law Review* (October, 1974), 925–954.

Levy, S. ETS and the "coaching" cover-up. *National ACAC Journal*, 1979, *23* (4), 14–21.

Rethwisch, B. P. & Fowler, G. Legal awareness in the college admissions process. *National ACAC Journal*, 1980, *24* (2), 8–11.

Shulman, C. H. *University admissions: Dilemma and potential.* Washington, DC: American Association for Higher Education, 1977.

The Regents of the University of California v. Bakke, 438, U.S., 265 (1978).

White, M. S. Psychological characteristics of the nurse practitioner. *Nursing Outlook*, 1975, *23* (3), 160–166.

5

Funding of
Primary Care Programs

Mary Fry Rapson

TYPES OF FUNDING

Primary care education programs can receive financial support from general fund allocations, fees or tuition, sales or royalties, investments and reserve funds. However, given the current trend in education toward budget retrenchment within an unstable economy, these funding allocations usually are not considered a firm base of support. Thus, it is often necessary for nurse practitioner educational and research programs to be funded extramurally from a variety of sources. The three main sources of external funding in the United States are governmental agencies, foundations, and business and industrial organizations. Vehicles frequently used by these institutions for financial support are grants, contracts, fellowships or traineeships, and free gifts.

Grants

Grants are given by the federal government as well as private foundations. They may provide funds for education, research, training, travel, construction, acquisition of equipment, or to supplement operating costs. The grant mechanism is usually flexible, based on broad goals and current priorities of the granting agency. Applicants have the freedom to design an approach to satisfy the specified agency goals and priorities. Grant funds are given for support of actual costs and are often dispersed geographically and program-matically. Federal grant programs are the direct result of congressional legislation and are announced in the *Federal Register*. Many training programs for primary care nurse practitioners and nurse midwives have been initially funded by the Department of Health and Human Services. Financial reports and final progress reports are required of grantees. Reporting requirements are minimal for foundations while detailed and extensive reporting is necessary for government grantees.

In addition to the federal government and foundations, many universities have seed-grant programs which may allocate small sums of money to help new faculty researchers launch individual research projects. These grants provide an excellent way of preparing for more formidable grant proposals from government and private industry.

Contracts

A contract is initiated by a federal agency or industrial corporation for a service or product based on specifications designed by the soliciting agency. These specifications usually determine the objectives, tasks, timetable, and procedure. Agency control and monitoring of performance are usually stricter with contracts than with grants in terms of reports, deadlines, specifications, and audits. Federal contract solicitations appear in the *Commerce Business Daily* (CBD). Frequently, academicians and health care professionals react negatively to contracts because they imply more control of performance than they would prefer. However, contracts need not be restrictive and frequently they are not. Contracts are usually awarded to the lowest bidder and include vigorous negotiations concerning the amount of money to be awarded. A danger to avoid is the temptation to underbid in time of financial need as the ultimate outcome may be negatively affected.

Fellowships and traineeships

Fellowships or traineeships are awards made to support advanced or continued education or research. Eligibility depends on many factors such as academic credentials, need, field of specialization, ethnic origin, and sex. Because of the expressed national need for more primary care services, many foundations, professional societies, and governmental agencies are providing funds for individual fellowships and traineeships in primary care nursing.

Gifts

Free gifts are often donated to human service organizations from alumni, civic groups, or businesses. These gifts are usually a sum of money for which no objectives are specified and no formal report need be made to the donor. The recipients of such gifts have flexibility when spending the money. However, this is the most difficult type of fund raising and should not be a substantive aspect of a primary care program. Free gift money can best be used to buy additional equipment, finance a short-term project, pay for travel, or continuing education needs of staff.

SOURCES OF INFORMATION ABOUT FUNDING

In order to fully explore the external funding opportunities for primary care nursing programs, it is necesary to set up a process of systematic data gathering. Most large agency or university settings have a grants management office whose primary purpose is to disseminate information about funding opportunities. The quality of services varies depending on the staff and its resources. The most helpful offices have a library which has standard references on all funding sources. If not, other excellent sources for information include libraries, workshops, newspapers, radio, television, government agencies, foundations, businesses, and "word-of-mouth". If a primary care educational program is serious about grant seeking, it may be useful to establish a library of its own on grantsmanship. One helpful reference for both public and private sources is the *Annual Register of Grant Support*. This book includes information on types of proposals accepted, deadlines, restrictions, and number of awards made in relationship to the number of applications received. Since the procedures for procuring information about federal sources, foundations, and local funding vary, each type will be discussed separately.

FEDERAL FUNDING

Obtaining adequate information about federal assistance programs is not easy. However, a number of references describing federal programs can be found in large libraries.

Catalog of Federal Domestic Assistance. This manual provides a comprehensive listing of all federal programs including eligibility, application, and deadline requirements. Addresses of regional and local federal offices are provided. It is indexed according to agency program, purposes, name of program, applicant eligibility, and subject. This publication is updated annually.

The Federal Register. The register provides daily information on federal programs including all proposed and finalized rules and regulations for legislation. It is published five days a week, Monday through Friday. Due dates for most grant applications are included and information is given on sources for more information about a selected grant.

Commerce Business Daily (CBD). The CBD announces contract bidding opportunities for procurement of goods and services. Every request for proposal (RFP) that exceeds $5000 must be published in this daily publication. The CBD is published every federal working day and includes notification of an RFP only once. There is usually short lead time and in some cases limited distribution of RFPs. Thus, conscientious contract seekers must study this document daily to keep abreast of the offerings. The funding agency's address and numerical codes needed for requesting the RFP are included in the document.

Request for Proposals (RFPs). RFPs are sent to institutions requesting them as well as to others who are known to be interested in the proposed contract. The RFPs include a description of the nature of work to be done as well as the exact specifications desired.

The United States Government Manual. This handbook is published by the federal government and describes every department and agency including addresses, telephone numbers, and names of key personnel. This book gives more in-depth information concerning each government agency than is given in the Catalog of Federal Domestic Assistance and is a good supplement to this publication.

Individual Agency Publications. Publications are disseminated by individual government agencies describing their programs and grant opportunities. Lists of governmental publications including individual subject areas can be obtained from the Government Printing Office.

FOUNDATIONS

While government agencies are mandated by law to provide the public information about their offerings, foundations are not. Thus, it is much more difficult to locate foundations, discover what they are interested in funding, and to elicit their interest in a project. Most foundations will provide individual copies of their annual reports upon request. These reports usually include a brief summary of their program priorities and past projects that were funded. For instance, a priority might be to fund pilot projects to give ambulatory care to inner-city adolescents. Relevant documents which assist in locating foundation funding are as follows:

The Foundation Directory. This publication lists private foundations and community trusts across the United States. The information is indexed by fields of interest, states, personnel names, and by foundation names. Descriptions include: name and address of the foundation, its donor, data and place of incorporation, purpose and activities, range of grants, and names of officers and trustees.

Foundation News. This is a bimonthly journal published by the Council on Foundations, Inc. It includes current information on foundation philanthropy of $5000 or more. Three listings are given: 1) by state, 2) by recipients, and 3) by key words or phrases.

The Foundation Grants Index Annual. Each yearly edition provides a list of grants made by the largest foundations in America. The amount of grant, name, location of recipient, description of the grant, and the grant identification number are described. By comparing yearly editions, it is sometimes possible to ascertain a pattern of funding exhibited by individual foundations.

Even with the use of these reference materials, it is very difficult to get a picture of the philanthropy of many of the foundations. The written materials are sometimes sketchy and goals are not stated clearly. Foundations do not usually want to receive long proposals or detailed inquiry letters. It is best to keep the initial letter to a single page which describes the project's importance to the foundation, the writer's qualifications, and the significance of the project to the applicant's organization and the health care community. A proposal should be no longer than two pages, be a concise summation, and include the estimated cost of the project. Foundations should be sought which have a particular interest in health care delivery, primary care, and/or nursing. If possible, try to speak with a board member, executive officer, or grants manager, or someone who has successfully obtained a grant from the foundation.

STATE, LOCAL, AND OTHER SOURCES

In searching for local funds, check with city and state governmental departments dealing with health and mental hygiene. Institutions of higher learning should be checked for recipients of state and local grants. They may be able to assist in obtaining information concerning grants sources. Newspapers and other media often announce grants from local governmental or business agencies. Regional professional organizations may have listings of funding opportunities for primary care related activities.

ASSESSMENT OF THE FUNDING ENVIRONMENT

Having identified potential sources of external funding, it is important to assess the applicant organization's programs, priorities, and funding environment as they relate to a grant application. When new funds are available, it is tempting to apply for those funds without considering how this project fits in with goals and priorities of the home institution. This type of decision making can lead to dire consequences. It is imperative that the effect of any new project be evaluated in terms of the effect on other programs within the institution, on staffing, on nonhuman resources, on existing funding, on consumers of the product or service, and other related variables.

It is also essential to know the extent to which funds are available in the applicant area or institution. This availability of funds is dependent on the state of the economy and on the competition for limited assistance. Nurse practitioners and primary care programs are still receiving priority funding from many governmental and private agencies even though the economic picture is not optimistic.

An assessment must be made in the home institution to determine the amount of support present for the grant application and how the institution will fare in a national or regional competition. Other organizations may have similar or better services, support of influential people, or a previous track record. It is important to evaluate the competition so that the writer can describe his unique approach in meeting an identified need which will be competitive. One way of being more competitive is to orient services to a target population. An example of this is offering primary care services to an underserved population or one that is receiving high priority in funding such as the elderly. Another approach is to turn potential competitors into collaborators by submitting a joint proposal. The latter commitment cannot be made lightly. Mutual collaboration may cause more problems than it solves in the long-term process.

Another important feature to consider is the extent of institutional and community support for the primary care issue. There may be total indifference, disagreement regarding definition of the problem, complete disapproval of the concept, or some forces not wanting primary care delivered at all. In some cases, there may be agreement concerning the problem but not in relation to the strategy for solving the problem. In designing a primary care grant proposal, clarification must be made concerning agreement, consensus, or indifference about the proposed project. When congruence is lacking, the proposal may receive great resistance within the community. Thus, careful grant planning includes assessment of the market conditions, relationships with competitors, congruence of project with the home institution, and an analysis of the issues involved.

APPLICATION FOR FUNDING

This phase begins when potential funding sources have been identified and the home institution's capability has been assessed. Deadline dates should be checked to ensure sufficient time to prepare and submit a worthwhile proposal. Time should be allowed to contact the potential funders to determine whether the funding source is interested in the proposal. Current information should be requested directly from the funding organization including guidelines, application forms, and other pertinent information. When all information is gathered, it should be read thoroughly, even the small print.

A relationship should be built with the funder long before the proposal is submitted. Calling the agency and keeping in touch with the right person may be all that is necessary. Many of the agency officials are willing to give comments on one or more preliminary drafts. The proposal is then written the way the funder wants it to be done. Even if the specific proposal is not funded initially, the relationships may continue to exist between the funding agency and the applicant. Frequently the latter is able to clarify future directions, assess current capacities, or learn technical information which will assist them to be more successful in the future.

The goal of the grant application is to submit a persuasive proposal—one that will convince the funders that the project is a good investment. The quality of the written proposal cannot be overestimated as the reviewers judge the anticipated value of the proposed project on the basis of the care and precision with which the application was prepared. The reviewers must be persuaded that:

1. The proposed project is within the scope of the objectives of the funding agency.
2. The proposed project is valuable because it will solve an immediate problem or add to existing knowledge.
3. The proposed project offers the opportunity to put a unique group of people to work on a problem that will never be more important than it is now.
4. The proposed project will produce important, concrete, and practical applications.
5. The proposed project has personnel that is acquainted with what has been done, is qualified to perform the described activity, and has access to the necessary resources to do so.
6. The proposed project offers results which sufficiently justify the time and money spent on it.

Once the project is accepted and funded, the proposal will serve as a promissory note, specifying the responsibilities assumed by the proposer in return for financial support. This does not mean that the proposal cannot be adapted to changing circumstances. However, it is a mistake to promise something impossible to deliver as the day of reckoning will come when the formal report is written.

PREPARATION OF THE PROPOSAL

Most funding agencies seek essentially the same information. Some use formats, others outlines, and still others specify no format at all. The design described in this chapter is a composite from several sources but bears the most similarity to expectations of federal agencies. A suggested outline is:

1. Title page(s)
2. Abstract
3. Project Narrative
   a. Introduction
   b. Problem Statement
   c. Objectives
   d. Methodology
   e. Evaluation of Objectives
4. Credentials of the Professional Staff
5. Budget
6. Future Funding and Plans for Continuation
7. Dissemination of Project Outcomes and Findings
8. References
9. Appendix

Title page

Most governmental agencies have their own forms for the title page. These forms must be filled out according to the funder's directions and failure to do so may mean rejection. The title page announces the project and provides information for identification purposes. Essential data should include title of the project, subject of the proposal, names and addresses of grantee organization and funding agency, project period, amount of money requested, signature of project director and other responsible people, an abstract, and date of submission.

The title of the project may be the first thing that strikes the reviewer's eye so it must be chosen with care. It should be brief, informative, creative, and written in lay language. A good way to develop a title is to elicit ideas from colleagues and staff.

Even though the title page is the first part of the proposal read by the reviewers, it is the last component to be prepared. The entire project must be written and ready for signatures before the title page can be finished.

The abstract

The abstract is a summary of the proposed project which gives the reviewers an overview in approximately 200 to 300 words. The abstract must capture the essence and tone of the project and motivate the reader to turn the page and read the body of the proposal. The abstract is written after the proposal is completed. Key points to cover are capabilities and accomplishments of the proposer, identified need, objectives, and proposed methodology to meet need, project addresses, costs of project, and the relationship of the project to the funding source's priorities.

The project narrative

The impact of the narrative system is dependent upon the value of the proposer's ideas and his or her abilities to state these concepts in concise, objective terms. Care should be taken to assure there is a logical flow from one section to another. Writing this section should be preceded by hours of thoughtful preparation. Before beginning the actual writing, it is helpful to develop an outline. This outline will serve as an organization tool as well as a mechanism to share ideas with administration who must give tentative approval before proceeding.

No one format for the narrative is suitable for all types of projects. However, the following components can be applied to most situations:

Introduction. The introduction is where credibility of the applicant organization is established. More often than not, proposals are funded on the basis of the reputation of the applicant organization or its personnel rather than on the merit of the project alone. Thus, it is imperative that the introduction inspires confidence that the proposal warrants consideration.

The introduction can be used to reinforce the relationship between the applicant organization's interests and those of the funding agency. Some information that can be presented is:

1. A succinct history of the organization.
2. Statistics documenting success in the field of interest.
3. Description of how this project fits into the goals of the organization.
4. Commendations by prominent individuals (letters of endorsement should be placed in the appendices).
5. Brief description of key staff.
6. Description of community involvement in the work.

The length of the introduction is proportional to the extent of the funding request. The more that is asked for, the more documentation that is needed to give proof of competence.

Problem/Need Statement. After introducing the applicant's capabilities and field of interest, the next challenge is to document the specific problems or needs that will be solved by the proposed project. The problem should be defined in terms that seem solvable with the proposed activity. Documentation should be provided regarding the problem's national and regional scope. Statistics and literature documentation are imperative. It is frequently helpful to compare the need in the applicant's area to that of another area, especially if there is competition geographically. It should be shown that this project is unique and is not duplicating others' efforts. Jargon and technical language should be avoided if possible. A logical connection should be made between the applicant organization's capabilities and the problems or needs proposed. The problem should be able to be accomplished by the applicant organization within a reasonable amount of time and resources.

Objectives. The problem statement should be logically developed so that it prepares the reader for the objectives. An objective is a specific, concrete, measurable outcome of a proposed project. They should be written in behavioral terms to avoid vagueness. The objectives should be realistic and achievable within the project framework. Well-written objectives are the key to successful proposals because they are directly linked with evaluation and imply good planning. When the objectives include standards of attainment and measurement criteria, the grantee can be held accountable for them by the funding officials. All granting agencies are looking for results.

Methodology. A detailed, step-by-step plan should be given in this section describing how the objectives will be met. There should be a presentation of techniques and procedures to be used; time estimates; instrumentation required; use of subjects; target population—subjects, control groups, or consumers; analysis of data; interpretation of results; resources needed; and extent of community involvement. In addition, funding officials may want to know why methods were chosen, their advantage to this project, whether they are cost-effective methods and whether the timing of these methods are realistic within the framework of the project. A description should be given regarding what personnel will be responsible for implementing each phase of the project. Professional jargon should be avoided. If used, it should be fully explained and/or defined. For instance, nurse practitioner and primary care should be operationally defined. Some reviewers reading the proposal may not be experts on the topic presented. The methodology section should be more detailed if it involves a research project rather than another type of activity. An education program should include a curriculum sequence and course outlines.

Evaluation of Objectives. The evaluation section is critical to a good proposal as it provides a mechanism for accountability and for improvement of a program. As stated previously, measurable objectives set standards for evaluation. A description should be given regarding how each objective will be measured; instruments to be used; evidence of accomplishment; and frequency of evaluation. If specific instrumentation has not been developed at the time of the proposal, plans should be included regarding selection or modification of tools.

Evaluation methodology should be as objective as possible.

Sometimes, an outside organization can conduct a more objective evaluation than is possible within the applicant organization. Otherwise, it should be clear who will be responsible for evaluation. The evaluation procedure should be ongoing, documenting change during progression of the project. One effective method of evaluation is a comparison of conditions before and after the proposed project. This is particularly useful if the change can be described in concrete terms such as a monetary savings in delivery of primary care education.

The real value of a good evaluation plan lies in conclusions drawn from the project results. Future project improvements are one of the things that funding officials are looking for in their grants. Thus, a description of the kinds of conclusions that might be drawn is helpful in the original proposal.

Credentials of the professional staff

This section should include the titles and qualifications of the professional staff, especially the project director. The biographical data should include professional training, experience, and achievements of the proposed staff. An emphasis should be made on the previous accomplishments of each staff member in the fields directly related to the project. If personnel are not identified at the time of the proposal, a description of duties, responsibilities, and qualifications expected should be given. The qualifications of the project director are critical and should be spelled out explicitly. Novice grant seekers can sometimes increase their chances of obtaining funding by securing collaboration with an established researcher, consultant, or other relevant worker. Where such a relationship has been established, the specific nature of this cooperation should be clarified. Use of consultants and research teams to bolster shortcomings in staff backgrounds can also be effective.

Budget

The budget section is often the most carefully scrutinized part of the proposal. It should represent a careful estimate of the financial needs to conduct the project. The anticipated costs are influenced by the needs of the project as well as by the limitations set by the granting agency. All budget items must be justified in the text of the proposal and comply with regulations of the funding agency and the applicant agency.

To prepare an accurate budget, information must be accumulated from a variety of sources. Grants office personnel or other financial experts can assist with this process. Another helpful source is an experienced colleague. It may be necessary to price such items as equipment, transportation, space rental, and so on, with the vendors themselves. Personnel offices can supply current data on salary rates and fringe benefits costs. There are many books available to assist the grantee with budget details and formats. However, it is wise to have a business manager or purchasing agent review the budget before submission of the proposal.

The grant applicant will be expected to differentiate between *direct* and *indirect* costs of the project. Direct costs are expenses which can be itemized and are incurred in conducting the project. Examples of these costs are salaries, supplies, equipment, travel, communications, publications, and books. Indirect costs are overhead expenses difficult to itemize on a project-to-project basis, for example, physical plant operation, library expenses, and utilities. These costs are calculated according to a negotiated formula between the granting agency and the applicant institution. The federal government usually sets a ceiling on the percentage of these costs allowed depending on the type of project. This amount is usually specified in the documents describing grant requirements.

Future funding and plans for continuation

This section presents a plan that will assure the funding agency that the project will be supported after the grant period is completed. Funders favor projects that need "start-up" money and have organizations which will financially support the program after the grant money is spent. An appropriate plan should include discussion of funding sources within the organization, fund raising methods available, degree of state or civic support, potential for future grants, and the need for a renewal grant. The more realistic the projections are, the more confident funding agencies will be in funding the project.

Dissemination of project outcomes and findings

Funding agencies are anxious that outcomes and findings be disseminated to interested parties. Thus, it enhances funding opportunities if a plan is given concerning dissemination of this information. Suggested dissemination techniques are:

1. Papers presented to national audiences.
2. An audio-visual presentation describing the project and its results.
3. Presentation of a workshop or seminar.
4. Journal articles on findings.
5. Published reports.
6. A project newsletter.
7. Press releases to local and national media.
8. Site visits for interested professions.

In addition to being advantageous to the granting agency, dissemination of project information is also a good public relations policy for the grantee organization. Evidence of media coverage of successful results makes future grant searching easier.

Appendix and references

The last two sections are the appendix and references. Three things should be included in the former category: items too long for the text; data that would influence the flow of the proposal; and information that documents assertions made in the body of the proposal. The reference section should include documents which substantiate the problem or need statement.

Organizational endorsement

Before the proposal can be submitted to a granting agency, the project director and appropriate institutional officials must sign the application. This endorsement implies commitment by the grantee institution to supply facilities and services to the project. If appropriate planning is done in advance with these officials, this step is a minor one. If agreement has not been reached, a significant delay could result in disqualification from the grant process. Since many grants have a short lead time, this phase of the application process takes considerable planning.

REVIEW AND PROCESS OF PROPOSAL BY FUNDING AGENCY

Applications submitted may be reviewed by staff members of the agency in addition to a review group with special expertise in the field. Sometimes the final decision is made by one agency head or a committee. Each agency has its own criteria for evaluation and is frequently willing to share with the potential grantee prior to submission of the proposal. Having this document is very helpful in preparing the proposal to ensure completeness and to demonstrate an awareness of expected standards. Possible evaluation criteria are: originality of concept; importance of the problem; relevance of the project to purposes of the funding agency; specificity of objectives, suitability of methodology, and evaluation of techniques; fiscal soundness; local support; technical merit; management potential; qualification of investigators; and institutional support.

Grant proposals can be rejected on the basis of content, writing style, flow, format, and mechanical mistakes. Attention should be given to making the proposal readable and to avoiding foolish technical errors. Common mistakes include a sloppy appearance, missed deadline, incomplete proposals, incorrect computations, fewer copies than requested by the funding agency, and failure to fulfill requirements for submission of a proposal. Many of these pitfalls can be eliminated by careful planning, review, and attention to detail.

Proposals found acceptable from a technical point of view are then reviewed from a budgetary standpoint. At this point, the funding official may enter into negotiations with the grantees regarding overall funding. During these discussions, the applicant has an opportunity to justify his position regarding budgetary requirements for the project. It is wise not to accept a reduction in budget unless a corresponding reduction in work is approved. After these discussions, the funding agency will make a decision regarding whether to grant the applicant his request and notify the proposer officially of the decision.

Even if proposals are rejected this process can be a productive experience. Most agencies will give written feedback to the applicant upon request regarding the reasons for rejection. In addition, the relationship established with individual granting officials during this proposal may be very beneficial in a future grant-seeking effort. Sometimes proposals must be resubmitted several times to be funded. If this is done, resubmission may be appropriate after yearly turnover of some of the reviewers has occurred.

If the primary care project is awarded a grant or contract, the work has just begun. The precision with which the proposal is designed will influence the ease of implementing the project. Good project management and report writing are essential in fulfilling funding agencies' expectations.

Ordinarily, obtaining external funding is a skill requiring considerable training and experience. It also requires a current knowledge of the sponsoring agencies, and their current policies and priorities. Understanding the major concepts of preparing a proposal coupled with the help of an experienced mentor will increase competence and effectiveness in obtaining funding for primary care nursing programs.

SUGGESTED READINGS

Abarbanel, K. The grantsmanship center: David and Goliath round two. *Foundation News*, 1978, *19*, (2), 21–23, 25–26, 28–29.

Barnard, R. Writing grant proposals. *Reflections*, 1980, *6*, (May-June), 8.

Campos, R. G. Acquiring foundation grants. *Journal of Nursing Administration*, June, 1980, *10*, (6), 16–23.

Caplovitz, D. The history of the inflation-recession proposal. *Grants Magazine*, 1978, *1*, (2), 166–170.

DeBakey, L. The persuasive proposal. *Foundation News*, 1977, *8*, (4), 19–27.

Decker, V. A. & Decker, L. E. *The funding process: Grantsmanship and proposal development*. Charlottesville, Virginia: Community Collaborators, 1978.

DesMarais, P. *How to get government grants*. New York: Public Service Materials Center, 1977.

Dixon, J. Developing the evaluation component of a grant application. *Nursing Outlook*, 1982, *30*, (2), 122–127.

Gortner, S. Research funding sources. *Western Journal of Nursing Research*. Spring, 1982, *4*, 248–50.

Hall, M. *Developing skills in proposal writing*, 2nd ed. Portland, Oregon: Continuing Education Publications, 1977.

Hennessey, P. The unique opportunity. *Grants Magazine*, 1978, *1*, (2), 170–176.

Jagger, J. How to write a research proposal. *Grants Magazine*, 1980, *3*, (4), 216–222.

Krathwohl, David. *How to prepare a research proposal*. 2nd ed. Syracuse, New York: School of Education, Syracuse University, 1976.

Lauffer, A. *Grantsmanship*. Beverly Hills, California: Sage Publications, 1977.

Lee, B. J. *Tips that make sense in grantsmanship*. New York: National League for Nursing, 1982.

Masterman, L. E. *The applicant's guide to successful grantsmanship*. New York: Hippocrene Books, Inc., 1978.

Orlich, D. C. & Orlich, P. R. *The art of writing successful R & D proposals*. Pleasantville, New York: Redgrave, 1977.

Reitman, J. E. *Grantsmanship: Money and how to get it*. Orange County, New Jersey: Marguis, 1978.

Sexton, D. L. Developing skills in grant writing. *Nursing Outlook*, 1982, *30*, (1), 31–38.

Teague, G. V. Request for a proposal: Solicitation for a federal contract. *Grants Magazine*, 1981, *4*, (1), 16–28.

White, V. P. *Grants: How to find out about them and what to do next*. New York: Plenum Press, 1975.

6

Curriculum Development

Despite hundreds of years of formalized teaching there is little definitive research concerning approaches to curriculum development. No one way of developing a program, course, or unit is demonstrably better than all others. In fact, the selection and sequencing of content has caused more discussion and occupied more meeting time than nearly any other issue in curriculum development. Developers of primary care nursing programs are no exception when they attempt to prepare a clinically competent practitioner who can deliver care within an organizational context.

Decision making for nurse practitioner curricula is in many ways a microcosm of larger educational issues. Should the learner be prepared to meet the immediate needs of society—a technological approach—or should he be prepared as a change agent to improve society and the profession? These choices become significant when the decision must be made whether to prepare graduates for the existing market or for a market they might create.

Many forces are at work in society and in educational settings to influence curricular decisions in primary care education. Some to consider are:

- geographic maldistribution of primary care providers
- nurse practice acts and related regulations

- accreditation standards
- certification requirements
- pool from which students are selected
- political climate
- economic conditions generally, and in health care particularly
- institutional support for the educational program
- quality of instructors available
- interprofessional support available

Some or all of these factors combine not only to influence the decision to begin a nurse practitioner program but how innovative it should be. In times of conservatism and decreased funding it will be more difficult to initiate new programs than during a period when change is encouraged and funded. However, one that meets an increasing need such as a geriatric program will receive support if it is well planned.

Those groups contemplating development of a nurse practitioner program are undoubtedly part of a larger educational or health care institution. Accordingly, this chapter is directed primarily toward nurse educators in established educational institutions. However, it is certainly possible for other institutions or groups to operate a program through providing continuing education as long as they adhere to standards of the accrediting bodies.

ACCREDITATION OF PROGRAMS

At the present time the American Nurses' Association (ANA) accredits continuing education programs that prepare for expanded roles as adult, pediatric, gerontologic, and family nurse practitioners. The National Association of Pediatric Nurse Associates and Practitioners (NAPNAP), in conjunction with the American Academy of Pediatrics, also accredits programs for pediatric nurse practitioners. The Nurses Association of the American College of Obstetrics and Gynecology (NAACOG) publishes guidelines for obstetric-gynecologic nurse practitioner programs. The National League for Nursing (NLN) accredits all nursing programs that award baccalaureate or higher degrees. There are no specific NLN criteria for expanded-role programs, but they must meet the overall criteria developed for schools of nursing (NLN, 1983). Nonetheless, it is wise for a college or university school of nursing to also adhere to the guidelines for short-term programs developed by other bodies such as ANA, NAPNAP, and NAACOG so that graduates may qualify to take certifying examinations. Usually it is possible to meet these guidelines in hours of didactic content. Clinical hours, if not adequate by the end of the collegiate program, can be supplemented with clinical experience after graduation. As new expanded roles emerge it can be expected that the current accrediting bodies and other interested groups will provide guidelines for program accreditation and offer certification examinations for graduates.

If nursing schools are interested in developing an undergraduate course or track in primary care nursing, many of the suggestions in this chapter will apply. Most nurse educators do not believe a fully qualified nurse practitioner can be prepared in a generic baccalaureate nursing program. (The NLN has recommended that nurse practitioners be educated at the master's level.) However, assessment skills and selected management skills basic to the nurse practitioner role can be integrated into undergraduate programs.

NEEDS ASSESSMENT

The need for the proposed program must be assessed much as one would survey the market when planning to manufacture a new product. Who will buy it? A survey of the potential market is in order. Here the analogy may fail because, in some aspects, the consumer of an expanded-role program is the student, but in other aspects the consumer is the medical profession, in that most nurses in expanded roles are employed by institutions. Data from both students and other professions are helpful. Survey of the physicians in the surrounding area or state can give valuable clues not only to the job market but also to sources of resistance or of support. Potential consumers of health care (potential patients) can also be surveyed to document the need for services nurse practitioners can provide. They can be queried directly through existing health care organizations, social or business groups, or through random mailings.

Any large survey will require a considerable outlay of human resources and funds. A small grant may be appropriate for this (see Chapter 5).

Other sources of data for a needs assessment of a regional or national scope are state and federal organizations such as the Institute of Medicine, The Center for Health Statistics, and the Bureau of Health Manpower of the Department of Health and Human Services, and state and local health departments. These groups gather statistics on the health needs of various populations in defined geographical areas and project the need for specialists as well as primary care providers. Although non-nursing organizations tend to view nurses in expanded roles as physician substitutes, their statistics can be combined with other sources for needs projections.

A final consideration in needs assessment is the interest of area nurses in preparing for an expanded role. This information is easily gathered through the present student body, alumni groups, and the local and state nurses' associations. Records of inquiries to the school may support the need for a new program.

RESOURCE ASSESSMENT

When the need for the new program is established, the adequacy of resources to support it are assessed. Support includes not only money and other concrete resources such as space, clinical and laboratory facilities, and salaries, but also expertise. Qualified nursing faculty is a requisite. Although early primary care nurse practitioner programs began with faculty only one step ahead of the students in skills acquisition, a larger pool of experienced nursing faculty is available now. In areas far from metropolitan medical centers it still may be necessary to send faculty away for a short course. Chapter 3 discusses the development and continuing education needs of nurse practitioner faculty. A thorough initial assessment of human resources will help identify the steps to be taken to develop competent nursing faculty. Faculty in existing departments can provide expertise without being fully qualified nurse practitioners. For instance, psychiatric faculty can teach the psychosomatic aspects of illness, and community health faculty can teach family assessment.

Indication of support from other professions and other institutions will strengthen the case for a new program, course, or track. Interviews with administrators in other schools and health care institutions often uncover expertise of potential use to a new program.

Projection should be made over a period of years for resources needed to support the program, not just for the short term. Assistance in developing resource needs and budget projections can be obtained from institutional administrators and business personnel. A comprehensive report on the feasibility of implementing the new program completes the needs and resource assessment phase. Chapter 5 discusses sources of funding for primary care educational programs.

CURRICULUM DESIGN

Curriculum has been defined as a process involving three steps: what one wishes to achieve (goal); how one wishes to achieve it (selection of learning experiences); and what one needs to know (the knowledge base) (Hoexter, 1976). The goals of the curriculum emanate explicitly or implicitly from the philosophy of the institution, school, or program. Consequently, the first step in developing a new program is to explore whether such a curriculum is consistent with any existing statement of philosophy or if one needs to be developed. According to Conley (1973), a philosophy reflects the beliefs of the faculty and explicates values and beliefs about the relationships of:

- the university to society and the universe
- nursing to the health care system
- the school of nursing to the university
- the school of nursing to the health care system

A similar operational definition of a philosophy can be developed for a component of a school of nursing or institution such as a hospital that might develop a program. For example, a relationship with society is implicit in the existence and functioning of a hospital.

A school of nursing proposing to begin an expanded-role program should examine the expressed philosophy of the total school and of the program (i.e., master's, baccalaureate) under which the new track or course is planned. Obvious discrepancies must be examined. To give an extreme and improbable example, a particular philosophy might imply only a dependent relationship of nursing with the health care system. This is obviously incompatible with the idea of the expanded nursing role. Most inconsistencies will be more subtle, or it may be impossible to decide because of vague or general language if a proposed program fits an existing philosophy. If the fit is not clear, these are cues that the faculty should reexamine and clarify the statement of philosophy. A concomitant benefit is that the faculty will be forced to examine the new program, thus exposing and hopefully confronting indecision or contradictions in philosophy.

When it is determined that the program is generally consistent with the philosophy of the institution, particularly in the beliefs about the role of the nurse in society, the philosophy for the primary care program is written. It should be derived from and consistent with the institutional philosophy at higher levels and should speak, at the least, to the place of the expanded role of nursing in society and to the faculty's belief about the potential learner. Most nurse practitioners and other expanded-role programs have focused principally on direct care but may additionally prepare graduates for leadership or change-agent roles in the health care system or for functional roles as administrators, teachers, or policy specialists.

The statement of philosophy should be concise and without undue use of academic or professional jargon. The content and meaning should be clear to a lay person outside the profession. "The philosophy provides a framework and guidelines for the development of objectives in the curriculum, the formulation of conceptual framework regarding the subject matter of nursing, and the identification of various instructional strategies for the implementation of the curriculum" (Conley, 1973, p. 13).

THE CONCEPTUAL FRAMEWORK

In addition to basing curriculum on philosophy and terminal behaviors (competencies), the approach, organizing principles, and sequencing of content are guided by the conceptual framework of the school or program. Chapter 1 discusses the importance of a nursing conceptual framework and suggests possibilities for the use of currently available frameworks for the teaching of primary care nursing. Nurses in expanded roles must be bilingual, that is, they must be familiar with the medical model to communicate with physicians but they must provide care through a nursing framework. A nursing focus may be provided in curriculum development through use of a particular framework or through the use of "threads" or concepts that offer continuity such as the nursing process, the wellness-illness continuum, or a systems approach. The framework or concepts serve as guides to organizing the curriculum and should be consistent with the philosophy. If a track or course in primary care is being planned, it too must fit into the philosophy of the school and program as well as contribute to the roles and functions of graduates. For instance, a developmental approach implies that curriculum content will be organized on an age (chronological) basis. This is often appropriate for a pediatric nurse practitioner program. A problem-oriented approach indicates that content is organized around the identification and management of client care problems.

When the statement of philosophy is agreed upon and a conceptual framework is chosen or developed, the task of curriculum development can proceed. First, a succinct look at how students learn is beneficial.

DOMAINS OF LEARNING

Bloom (1977) divided learning into three domains: cognitive, affective, and psychomotor. A hierarchy of complexity of objectives in each domain was also identified.

The cognitive domain is that area of learning that emphasizes memory of content and its reproduction. The affective domain is that learning expressed as feeling tones, emotions, attitudes, interests, or values. The psychomotor domain is concerned with motor control, manipulation of objects, or acts requiring neuromuscular coordination. Detailed hierarchical taxonomies were developed for the cognitive and affective domains (Bloom, 1977; Krathwohl, Bloom, & Masea, 1969). Cognitive learning can vary from being able to simply recall a fact, to application or analysis, and finally to synthesis and evaluation at the highest levels. The accomplishment of affective learning is demonstrated on a continuum of attending (being sensitized), responding, valuing, organizing values, and finally, by having a value complex. At the highest affective level, a student selectively responds consistent with an internal set of values.

Cognitive learning represents the majority of formal learning and is addressed in many books and articles. More recent interest has developed in the affective domain. Certainly, attitudes and values are critical to high-level functioning in a human services profession. The autonomy and accountability inherent in expanded roles requires attention to development of affective behavior. For instance, a practitioner may need to help patients make decisions between treatment modalities.

In a particular area of affective learning, Kohlberg (1969) has sparked a great interest in moral development. Although much of his work pertains to children, his levels of moral reasoning are applicable to adults and specifically to nurses. Undoubtedly, the difficulties in measuring the attainment of affective learning constrains nursing faculty from including it in expectations of students. Yet it is often apparent when a student does not have values or a "philosophy" consistent with role expectations. This is even more crucial in a new area such as primary care where attitudes and values of one nurse practitioner may be ascribed to a whole class or group. Affective learning is inexorably linked to cognitive and psychomotor learning in that attitudes and interests determine motivation to learn. In an even larger context, a value complex that values learning is necessary for a successful education experience.

Bloom did not speak to psychomotor objectives. However, Fitts and Posner (1979) provided valuable insight into the learning of skills. They delineated two broad classes of skill learning—perceptual motor and language. Perceptual motor skills are further broken down into gross body skills, manipulative skills, and perceptual skills.

Because expanded roles entail learning of perceptual motor skills new to many nurses, it is worthwhile to explore the phases of learning skills further. According to Fitts and Posner, skill learning is hierarchical and sequential. First, the beginner in an adult skill-learning situation must understand the task and what it demands. This is called the early or cognitive phase. In the intermediate or associative phase, old habits and errors in performance are eliminated. Proper scheduling of practice and sequencing of the components of the skill are important here. In the final or autonomous phase, skill performance is less subject to cognitive control and requires less processing. The application of information about skills learning to psychomotor tasks required of nurse practitioners and other "hands-on" providers is discussed in Chapter 8. References on learning principles and theories are listed at the end of this chapter.

AN APPROACH TO CURRICULUM DEVELOPMENT

The principle of "working backward" is important, and the remainder of this chapter is organized around that principle. It forces the planner to focus on the final product which here is a competent practitioner. The potpourri approach of starting with beginning competencies and working forward by patching together segments of content to make a unit, units to make a course, and courses to make a program loses sight of the goal and encourages instructors to include and protect their own pet bit of content.

Throughout the process of program development the curriculum planner must ask what capability the learner must have to perform a task or acquire a body of knowledge successfully. A psychomotor task such as the cardiac examination requires a knowledge of cardiovascular functioning. Giving anticipatory guidance to a parent requires knowledge of growth and development.

In the process outlined in Figure 6-1 curriculum planners must assure that each content level contributes to the making of the graduate. The program objectives are a bridge between entering knowledge and skills and terminal behaviors. The admissions standards discussed in Chapter 4 set the initial level of expected performance.

Terminal objectives

The first step in curriculum development is to describe the roles and functions of the nurse who completes the program or course in the form of program objectives. These are known as terminal objectives and describe the behaviors or competencies the student should

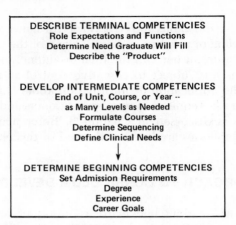

Figure 6–1. Sequence of Program Development

demonstrate at the end of the program as a beginning practitioner. These are usually stated in global terms such as, "diagnoses and plans treatment of patient with stable health problems" or "screens school-age children for learning problem."

Intermediate objectives

Intermediate objectives are then developed. In a master's program these are the semester or course end objectives. In a continuing education program or a course in primary care these may be end-of-unit objectives. In reality, there can be one or several levels of intermediate objectives—whatever is necessary to delineate the components needed. They serve as markers for the student's progress from initial competencies to terminal behaviors. Some principles and techniques of writing objectives should be considered before proceeding to course development.

Writing instructional objectives

Nurse educators have wholeheartedly endorsed the use of instructional objectives to specify desired outcomes. In fact, there is sometimes a tendency to become too specific and detailed in the enthusiasm to write in behavioral terms. Nonetheless, the goal of education is modification of behavior, and the practice of delineating desired behaviors of the students at the end of segments of instruction provides the basis on which achievement can be measured. Some objectives give the student guidance in deciding the areas to emphasize when studying. Terminal and course-end objectives also indicate the purpose of the course and help students decide the suitability of a particular program or course for them. Another benefit for the instructor is that, by listing all learning objectives, the time and other resources needed to teach the content should become apparent.

Some general points can be made about the writing of instructional objectives. The following suggestions were compiled from sources both in general education and in nursing.

1. An "ideal" objective should contain
    a. a statement of what the learner is expected to be able to do;
    b. the important conditions under which the performance is to occur; and
    c. the criteria of acceptable performance. (Mager, 1975)
2. The degree of specificity should be appropriate. Objectives for a particular class are more specific than for course objectives which are still more specific than program objectives.
3. Objectives should be stated in terms of behavior that can be observed and/or measured. Verbs must be chosen that have few interpretations. For example, "to compare" is much more specific than "to understand."
4. The level of expectation in an objective should be appropriate for the level of student and for the particular placement in the course or program. For instance, students in a beginning physical assessment course can be expected to "state" or "identify" in a cognitive learning experience or to understand a complex psychomotor task. Near the end of the program, particularly a graduate program, synthesis of cognitive knowledge and proficient practice of psychomotor skills in some areas are not unreasonable expectations.
5. A corollary to number 4 is that instructional objectives at each level should feed into the next higher level and become more complex as the student progresses through the course or program.
6. Objectives should be attainable within the program and capable of being measured.

Examples for different programs

Several examples of leveling of objectives are given in the following figures. A decimal system helps define the levels of objectives. Table 6-1 demonstrates some of the beginning and intermediate competencies needed to achieve a terminal objective in a master's

Table 6-1. Example of Leveled Objectives in a Master's Nurse Practitioner Program

The student will be able to:

1.0   *Provide health care to clients with stable, chronic problems.

1.1   **Describe the multiple etiologies, and signs and symptoms of selected health problems.

1.1.1   ***Describe the etiology, signs and symptoms of hypertension.

1.1.2   ***Identify the secondary causes of hypertension.

BEGINNING COMPETENCY   Demonstrate a knowledge of basic physiology of the cardiovascular system.

1.2   **Apply epidemiological and statistical principles to the identification of major chronic health problems.
1.2.1   ***Identify risk factors that predispose to the development of hypertension.
1.2.2   ***Compare the incidence of essential hypertension to that due to secondary causes.

BEGINNING COMPETENCY   Define the terms - - risk factor, incidence, prevalence. Relate the incidence of hypertension in the U.S.

Key

*   Terminal objective
**   First-level objective
***   Second-level objective

Table 6-1. (*continued*)

1.3	**Evaluate the health status of a client with an elevated blood pressure.
1.3.1	***Perform a complete cardiovascular exam.
1.3.2	**Identify health practices that are related to the development of hypertension.

| BEGINNING COMPETENCY | Take a blood pressure accurately. Distinguish normal from abnormal heart sounds. |

1.4	**Provide health care for patients with hypertension.
1.4.1	***Counsel hypertensive patients on proper nutrition.
1.4.2	***Monitor efficacy and side effects of medications.

| BEGINNING COMPETENCY | Describe the actions and side effects of the major antihypertensive drugs. Describe one stress reduction technique. |

Key

| ** | First-level objective |
| *** | Second-level objective |

---

program that prepares adult primary care nurse practitioners. Master's programs have other curricular elements such as research, statistics, cognates, and nursing theory. It is quite legitimate to ask the student to apply, analyze, or synthesize knowledge from other courses in a clinical course providing that the content was in a prerequisite course. In a certificate course that is concentrated in a few months, some prerequisite basic and applied science content is integrated into clinical courses. How much is determined by the required level of knowledge at entrance to the program.

Table 6-2 begins with a terminal objective for a certificate program to prepare pediatric nurse practitioners. Nurses with a diploma and two years' pediatric experience may enter this program.

Table 6-3 illustrates the progress toward a terminal objective for a course in physical assessment for seniors in a baccalaureate nursing program. This table also demonstrates that cognitive and psychomotor intermediate objectives may be needed to achieve a general terminal objective.

Table 6-4 develops objectives in the affective domain that are pertinent to the nurse practitioner role. A timetable is more difficult to establish with this domain, and levels of objectives may be skipped when a student gains sudden insight or has experiences that force values clarification.

COURSE DEVELOPMENT:
THE ART OF SEQUENCING

Much valuable time and energy can be spent debating the merits of one pattern of content sequencing versus another both within and across courses. The goals of ordering or sequencing are to teach content in the most meaningful and the most efficient manner. These goals are not always compatible, and limitation of resources—including time—may determine that efficiency must win out over meaningfulness. Some sequencing decisions are obvious. Others are chicken and egg issues, but the vast majority of decisions can be made by using the philosophy, terminal objectives, and conceptual framework as a basis. The amount of content in a course must be compatible with credit given and the logical division of content as determined by the faculty. The major concepts are used as organizing themes. For instance, the nursing process is a common concept that becomes a curricular theme. Even more helpful, the nursing process contains sequential subconcepts: assessment, planning, implementation, and evaluation. A nurse practitioner program using the nursing process as a major concept might plan a first course on assessment only, then proceed through one or more courses to teach the re-

Table 6-2. Example of a Leveled Objective in a Continuing Education Program for Pediatric Nurse Practitioners

---

The student will be able to:

1.0	*Provide well-child care for children from birth to 18 years.
1.1	**Provide well-baby care for infants from birth to 1 year.
1.1.1	***Elicit and record a pregnancy and birth history.
1.1.2	***Perform a physical examination to identify abnormalities.
1.1.3	***Obtain a food intake history.
1.1.4	***Evaluate the parent-infant relationship.
1.1.5	***Give anticipatory guidance on physical, physiological, and developmental needs of the infant.
1.2	**Demonstrate a knowledge of the developmental tasks of infants and children.
1.2.1	***Discuss the sequence of motor maturation in infants.
1.2.2	***Relate the role of stimulation in infant development.

BEGINNING COMPETENCIES

Describe the importance of the mother-infant relationship.
Define — bonding, attachment, separation behavior.
Demonstrate a knowledge of: common problems in infancy; the normal birth process.

Key

*	Terminal objective
**	First-level objective
***	Second-level objective

99

Table 6-3. Example of a Leveled Objective in a Physical Assessment Course for Baccalaureate Students

---

The student will be able to:

1.0	*Perform a thorough assessment of the chest, distinguishing normal from abnormal findings.
1.1	**Describe the normal shape of the chest wall.
1.2	**Identify the signs of respiratory distress.
1.3	**Percuss the chest wall, describing areas of resonancy, hyperresonancy, and dullness.
1.4	**Auscultate the chest for areas of vesicular, bronchial, and bronchovesicular sounds.

BEGINNING COMPETENCIES	Identify major landmarks of the chest. Describe the events of the respiratory cycle. Demonstrate proper use of the stethoscope.

Key

*	Terminal objective
**	Intermediate objective

---

maining subconcepts. The similarities and differences of the nursing process and the sequencing of diagnosis and management using the medical model have not escaped the recognition of nurse practitioners. They both stem from the general problem-solving process. The differences lie in the content taught under each subconcept that is unique to either nursing or medicine.

Other concepts that guide sequencing are wellness-illness, simple to complex, a developmental perspective, or by practice setting (hospital, ambulatory, community). Tyler (1969) suggested that three criteria should be used in organizing curriculum: continuity, se-

Table 6–4. Leveling of Affective Objectives

The student:

1.0 *Values the contributions made by nurse practitioners to health care delivery.

1.1 **Recognizes the contribution of nursing to total health care.

1.2 **Offers evidence from literature supporting competencies of nurse practitioners.

1.3 **Volunteers services at a health fair or other community project.

2.0 *Develops plan of care recognizing cultural differences in child care practices.

2.1 **Describes family roles and functions in various cultures.

2.2 **Appreciates historical background for differences in child care practices.

2.3 **Counsels parents in a nonjudgmental manner.

2.3.1 ***Selects alternatives culturally acceptable to parents.

Key

*   Terminal objective
**   First-level objective
*** Second-level objective

quence, and integration. Continuity is the chronological sequencing of major curricular elements. Sequence, in Tyler's usage, refers to the building of each step on preceding learning. Integration is the organization of learning so that the student generalizes new knowledge to other courses and other situations. Several authors caution that many students do not learn in a "logical" sequence and that the instructor should assess how each student learns. Some typical organizing schemes can be evaluated in light of the previous discussion on learning and the characteristics of nursing.

Simple to complex learning

Learning of concepts, subconcepts, and psychomotor skills involve different types and levels of learning. Proceeding from simple to more complex forms of learning is one organizing scheme for both course placement and individual learning experiences. Gagne (1965) proposed a hierarchy of eight types of learning.

1. Signal learning
2. Stimulus-response learning
3. Chaining
4. Verbal association
5. Discrimination learning
6. Concept learning
7. Rule learning (relationship among concepts)
8. Problem solving.

Although providing health care involves the highest level of problem-solving skill, the components of any specific patient-nurse practitioner contact may involve several lower levels of learning. For example, the diagnosis of a rash on the wrist of a 20-year-old woman may include *verbally associating* words such as red-raised-irregular border. The *discrimination* of the characteristics of these lesions from all others the student has seen is the next step. The next is the recognition of the *concept*, "rash," as a class of dermatological lesions. These steps undoubtedly occurred very early in the student's life and before any professional training. An example of *rule learning* in this clinical situation is the rule that rashes due to allergies usually itch. It is at this level that some knowledge is brought from the basic nursing education but more must be added to reach the highest cognitive level of *problem solving*. More rules are added such as: (1) people who are outdoors may touch poison ivy, or (2) people may be allergic to metal in jewelry.

The difficult part of applying known rules to problem solving in clinical situations is the qualifier in the rule—sometimes, maybe, probably. The tentativeness of rules in human care is difficult for some students to accept and illustrates the interplay of affective and cognitive learning. Until the student accepts and appreciates the tentativeness and ambiguity of certain rules, it is difficult to apply problem-solving techniques to human problems. A teaching technique used to encourage this appreciation is to ask the student to prioritize possible diagnoses. The concept of probability versus trial and error guessing is essential to the learning of clinical problem solving.

Body systems

Body systems is the organizing scheme for traditional medical education. There are pros and cons to organizing assessment and management courses around this scheme. On the positive side, it is familiar to most health professionals, is concrete, and needs little explication before proceeding to content. However, there are many negative aspects to this approach. Most obvious is the lack of an integrating scheme or a holistic view of human beings, a foundational concept in nursing. Using body systems to teach assessment and management in the traditional way usually violates any attempt to move from the simple to complex in that most complex systems of the head and neck are taught first.

Developmental stages

Sequencing of content for part or all of a program by developmental stages is rational, particularly if development throughout the life cycle is part of the philosophy and conceptual framework. Most pediatric programs for basic and advanced nursing programs use this scheme. It is particularly appropriate when teaching about the health promotion needs of clients of all ages.

For teaching the assessment and management of particular health problems this scheme may not be efficient or effective. For example, a particular health problem such as anxiety and depression may have manifestations at several age levels. If the content is taught at each age level, the student may not get a coherent picture of the course of the problem and content is unnecessarily retaught.

Sequencing for part-time study

With a decrease in external funding and an increase in tuition costs, special attention must be given to problems of sequencing of courses for part-time graduate students. It is helpful for student advisement to lay out several possible part-time programs. Some students who work fulltime may be able to take 4-6 credit hours per semester. Others may choose deliberately to study half-time because of family or other needs. Generally, it is more beneficial to take the supportive conceptual and cognitive content such as courses in physiology and health care systems first. Because psychomotor learning and role acquisition benefit from continuity, courses in diagnosis and management should be grouped together. Care must be taken in advising the student so that needed courses are available near the end of the program and in the proper sequence. For example, a student may need only two courses to graduate but discover there is only one section of each exactly at the same hours. Or a prerequisite course might be available only every other semester.

SUMMARY

The development of expanded-role programs should not be undertaken until a thorough needs assessment is completed. Many forces influence both the decision to start a new program and the content it should include. In approaching the task of designing a curriculum, these forces as well as sound educational practice must be considered.

Development of objectives should proceed "backward," that is, the students' competencies at the end of the program or course must be described in behavioral terms first. Then intermediate objectives are developed. The sequencing of courses and content within courses should be based on some predetermined concept that follows logically from the philosophy of the program and is consonant with learning theories. Some flexibility of course sequencing should be provided for part-time students in collegiate programs.

REFERENCES

Bloom, B. S. (Ed.). *Taxonomy of educational objectives. Handbook I: Cognitive domain.* New York: Longmans, Inc., 1977.

Conley, V. C. *Curriculum and instruction in nursing.* Boston: Little, Brown and Company, 1973.

Fitts, P. M. & Posner, M. I. *Human performance.* Westport, Connecticut: Greenwood Press, 1979.

Gagne, R. M. *The conditions of learning.* New York: Holt, Rinehart and Winston, 1965.

Hoexter, J. The purposes and approaches in selecting and organizing curriculum content and learning experiences. In *Curriculum in graduate education in nursing, Part II: Components in the curriculum development process.* New York: National League for Nursing, 1-9, 1976.

Kohlberg, L. Stage and sequence: The cognitive developmental approach to socialization. In D. A. Goslin (Ed.), *Handbook of socialization theory and research.* Chicago: Rand McNally, 1969, 347-380.

Krathwohl, D. R., Bloom, B. S. & Masea, B. B. *Taxonomy of educational objectives. Handbook II: Affective domain.* New York: Longmans, Inc., 1969.

Mager, R. F. *Preparing instructional objectives,* 2nd ed., 1975.

National League for Nursing. *Criteria for the appraisal of baccalaureate and higher degree programs in nursing,* 5th ed. New York: National League for Nursing, 1983.

Tyler, R. W. *Basic principles of curriculum and instruction.* Chicago: University of Chicago Press, 1969.

SUGGESTED READINGS

American Nurses' Association. *Accreditation of continuing education in nursing.* New York: American Nurses' Association, 1975.

American Nurses' Association. *Guidelines for short-term continuing education programs preparing adult and family nurse practitioners.* New York: American Nurses' Association, 1975.

American Nurses' Association. *Directory of accredited organizations, approved programs/offerings and accredited non-degree granting expanded role programs in nursing.* New York: American Nurses' Association, 1978.

Bevis, E. O. *Curriculum building in nursing: A process,* 3rd ed. Saint Louis: C. V. Mosby Company, 1982.

Holt, F. M. The primary care nurse practitioner role. In *Developing the functional role in master's education in nursing.* New York: National League for Nursing, 1980.

Huckabay, L. M. D. *Conditions of learning and instruction in nursing.* Saint Louis: C. V. Mosby Company, 1980.

Kapfer, M. B. *Behavioral objectives in curriculum development: Selected readings and bibliography.* Englewood Cliffs, New Jersey: Educational Technology Publications, 1971.

Lindvall, C. M. (Ed.). *Defining educational objectives.* Pittsburgh: University of Pittsburgh Press, 1964.

National League for Nursing. *Faculty-curriculum development, Part I: The process of curriculum development.* New York: National League for Nursing, 1974.

National League for Nursing. *Course development in schools of nursing.* New York: National League for Nursing, 1982.

Reilly, D. E. & Phaneuf, M. C. *Behavioral objectives in nursing: Evaluation of learner attainment.* New York: Appleton-Century-Crofts, 1975.

Schweer, J. E. (Ed.). *Defining behavioral objectives for continuing education offerings in nursing: A four level taxonomy.* Thorofore, New Jersey: Charles B. Slack, 1981.

7

Teaching Didactic Content: The Classroom Experience

It is not the intent of this chapter to suggest *what* should be taught. That is determined by the program or course objectives. Specific content is then developed using the process outlined in the previous chapter. Rather, this chapter includes *how* didactic content in primary care can be taught through classroom activities and assignments.

What is best taught in the classroom? Generally, knowledge that is in the cognitive domain is transmitted most effectively in a formal teaching situation. Affective learning will also take place through the attitudes conveyed consciously or incidentally by the instructor.

The level of cognitive knowledge required depends on the specific content of the course and the level of the student. In a continuing education program to prepare nurse practitioners, content moves rapidly from low levels based on Bloom's taxonomy (1977) (identify, recall) to higher levels where students are required to apply, synthesize, or evaluate content. Students learning health assessment in a baccalaureate nursing program are not expected to manage illness care independently but should be able to do history-taking, perform a physical examination, and identify health needs. In this case, emphasis is on Bloom's level of comparing and contrasting normal and abnormal findings. In a master's program that prepares nurse practitioners, students can reasonably be expected to develop a substantial amount of high-level cognitive knowledge. They should be able to apply and synthesize learning from previous and concurrent courses. For example, if the subject of the class is management of asthma in children, knowledge in such diverse areas as developmental psychology, parent teaching, community resources, and lung physiology is applied when making management decisions. The classroom teacher, by the skillful use of well-chosen methods, can facilitate application and synthesis of knowledge from several specialties to the topic under consideration.

Instructional methods to be considered in this chapter are: (1) lecture; (2) discussion; (3) seminars; (4) panel discussion; and (5) the use of audiovisual media. Teaching techniques that are less widely used are discussed in Chapter 9. These include techniques such as classroom role-playing, simulations through the use of games, computer programs, and professional patients. Following the discussion of general teaching methods, the use of texts, library materials, and other assignments are considered. Finally, some approaches to assist student learning are examined.

GENERAL CONSIDERATIONS

When choosing a classroom teaching method, several factors are involved. First, it is recognized that no one method is superior to all others. Each has special but not unique advantages. Some teachers are only comfortable with certain methods. For example, if a person is ill at ease when speaking formally to large groups, use of media and small discussion groups are a better choice. On the other hand, some teachers have the gift of enthralling a large number of students in a two-hour lecture using little more than a piece of chalk and their own resourcefulness. For the latter, lectures or lectures and discussion are the methods of choice.

The cost of different methods is important as funding for educational programs decreases. Some multimedia techniques motivate and hold students' interest but are initially much more expensive than a lecture. Some combinations of methods are synergistic; others are repetitious and consequently costly. Preparation time for methods will vary widely and is another factor to consider in assessing cost.

The nature of the student population is another variable to consider in the choice of teaching method. The use of a motion picture in the classroom is no longer a major event for urban-reared young students. Novelty using media will be difficult to achieve as more homes have video recorders, slide projectors, and other new communication technologies. We are in a gadget-oriented era; it is quite possible that in a few years students will value the novel opportunity to hear live lectures and to discuss problems with clinicians. Computer-assisted learning will be less threatening to the young student who grows up with a home computer, whereas a student with no previous computer contact may concentrate so much on gaining access to the program that the value of the experience is lost.

Instructors are loathe to change teaching methods, especially if they must give up one proven by time to be effective. This is only human nature, but a good teacher looks for ways to continually improve and invigorate instruction. Experimentation revitalizes content taught several times and renews instructor interest as well. This is not to advocate change for change's sake, but to suggest that preparation for new roles deserves the most effective teaching methods available.

The balance of various methods in teaching didactic content varies according to content and level of student. More advanced students can be expected to engage in self-study activities, so that less lecture and more discussion and seminars are used. Beginning students need reinforcement and reteaching by different methods. For them, more lecture to ensure the teaching of critical content is necessary. More than three or four lecture hours per week per course in a baccalaureate or master's program is burdensome for teachers and students and may indicate a need to divide the course. In a continuing education course that is full-time and contains both clinical and didactic, no more than three to four hours per day should be pure lecture. Students are unable to prepare properly for more lectures and soon fall behind.

Most often, the nature of the content largely determines the teaching method. Conley (1973, p. 488) states that methods should follow, not dictate, teaching aims. There is often more than one method from which to choose. As methods are considered on the following pages, advantages, disadvantages, skills and materials needed, and tips on use in primary care are discussed where appropriate.

LECTURE

At first examination, it would seem that the lecture method is the place to impart facts—and this is the way it is used by far too many teachers. Actually, the printed word, for example, texts, handouts, and articles, is a much better vehicle for presenting factual material than lectures. Lecturing was the original method of group teaching before the printing press was invented. Perhaps because of this, it has persisted in spite of the availability of more economical methods of dispensing facts. The reasons for popularity of lectures are numerous and of only peripheral interest. Undoubtedly, the quantifiable nature of the process, that is, the ability to count hours in the classroom, numbers of students, and student-teacher ratios is the underlying reason for the persistence of the lecture method.

If lecturing is not a good method for teaching facts, what are its uses? McKeachie (1978, p. 31) states that live lecturing is most effective where there are considerable variations among students in ability, relevant background, or motivation and where feedback to the lecturer is important. Certainly, the diversity of backgrounds in nursing education and experience meets his first criterion. The best uses of the lecture are to help students develop and apply concepts, practice problem-solving skills, and generalize knowledge already learned. Students are not passive in lectures. Feedback is given through both verbal and nonverbal behavior that the lecturer must recognize. A look of puzzlement or tentative raising of hands are signals that the lecturer is either moving too fast or the message is unclear. In addition, students are actively learning by making new associations, developing hunches, evaluating previous learning, and categorizing new concepts. A few succinct examples from the lecturer can trigger a sudden insight (often called an *aha!* experience) where previously isolated bits of learning come together on a conceptual level. Lectures can be used to exchange information, clarify concepts, and stimulate further study.

Although it is possible to deliver a didactic lecture to any size of student group, in nursing this method is most often combined with other methods either to give or receive information. Most classes for nurse practitioner or midwifery students are composed of twenty students or less—a good size for integrating lecture with discussions, panels, and individual reports. Media can be a welcome diversion in a two-hour lecture. Discussion as a total group or in "buzz" sessions can be used to identify fuzzy areas, misunderstandings, and other blocks to learning inherent in lecturing to a large group. Eble (1976) states that "the enemy of learning is primarily other learning" (p. 4). In learning an expanded role especially, previous knowledge or deep-seated attitudes may prevent or delay new conceptualizing unless dealt with early. As a simple example, ideas about the concept of primary nursing may interfere with learning the concept of primary care nursing. Combining discussion with lecture may identify difficulties students have with new knowledge. Straight lecture is not appropriate for professional issues or any content that should result in attitude changes.

Skills needed

An instructor must have extensive knowledge of the subject matter to deliver an authoritative lecture. A class presenting a concept for practice that is developed strictly from library research will lack the authenticity of one supported by the teacher's own experience. A nursing instructor may be forced to decide between spending many hours researching a new topic to assure that the content is up to date or inviting a guest lecturer with "hands-on" experience but who is inept at lecturing. The ideal lecturer, of course, is one who knows the subject well and who can deliver an organized and lively talk. Lecturers do not all have to be qualified nurse practitioners because content from other areas of nursing are appropriate for expanded-role programs. Community health faculty can teach family assessment, psychiatric faculty can teach the psychologic aspects of illness and health, and medical-surgical faculty can teach the pathophysiology of diseases within their expertise. In addition to being competent however, they should be knowledgeable and supportive of the expanded role students are assuming.

Even an expert clinician will require an inordinate amount of time preparing a class if the content is highly technical. Exhaustive reading submerges the teacher in the subject. A computerized literature search combined with scanning of current journals is helpful in finding up-to-date sources. This will assure that information is current, especially if the subject is in a rapidly changing area. Such a search also identifies the most applicable readings for student assignments. Nursing and medical indexes can be used to identify the best and most recent references.

The development of lesson plans where objectives, content, assignment, activities, and evaluation methods are listed organizes the lecture for the teacher. A briefer outline can be given to the students. Veteran lecturers know that to keep the attention of some students, some important bits of information should be kept for presentation during the lecture rather than being assigned. This can be content such as a new diagnostic test, a mode of treatment, or an unusual case history.

Assignments should be made sufficiently ahead of a lecture to assure adequate preparation. Copies of articles can be made available through the library or the instructor. Nothing is more frustrating to a student than to have required reading assigned from obscure journals that are not available in their institution. Most students do need instruction in using library and other resources, and an orientation to learning resources should be scheduled early in a program.

Efforts should be made to have an inviting and attractive classroom. Many programs use the same classroom throughout a course so that learning aids can be left in the room or on the walls. Anatomical charts or algorithms are helpful when teaching specific content. Attendance to proper climate control and comfort in seating will pay off in increased attention span and motivation. Media hardware should be available on time and in working order and copies of handouts ready.

Tips on successful use of the lecture

There are perhaps more "don'ts" than "do's" in the literature on lecturing. Eble (1976) warns, "don't lecture," but talk and converse (p. 42). Equally emphatic is "don't read your notes." Even with adequate preparation, attention to the environment, and a motivated student group, teaching is a performing art. Rather than making a conscious attempt to be impersonal, dispassionate, and totally objective, the personality of the speaker should come through. "Human beings interest other human beings" (Eble, 1976, p. 12). Further he insists that:

> Few subjects are value-free, and honesty about where one stands, illumination about how one has arrived there, and respect for the beliefs of others form a better basis for teaching than does a resolute, ultimately dogmatic posture of impersonal objectivity. (p. 3)

A passionate commitment to expanded roles in nursing coupled with an abiding belief in students' ability to learn and perform motivates students to put forth more effort and promotes self-confidence. There are many issues concerning expanded roles and patient management that are controversial and lend themselves to the expression of opinions, and analysis of how the lecturer arrived at them. This stance may be alien to some nursing instructors who equate sterility of style with academic objectivity. It appears self-evident that in teaching others to care for human beings, part of role modeling is in revealing some of our own humanity to students. In this regard, humor can be used naturally and judiciously to increase the rapport between lecturer and students.

The lecturer should (1) "tell them what you're going to tell them; (2) tell them; then (3) tell them what you've told them" (McKeachie, 1978, p. 33). If two conflicting viewpoints are given, the first one presented leaves the most impression. An application of this phenomenon is the presentation of several possible treatments for a given patient problem. Students will tend to remember the first presented so it should be the one the lecturer wants to dominate, rather than less effective modes. In pharmacology, for instance, first-level drugs should be emphasized. In assessing the children's growth and development, the most common tools should be presented first and in greater detail than those less commonly used.

Most new teachers try to include too much in a class period. Having thirty minutes of material ready will probably fill a fifty-minute period. Additional examples or case studies can be ready for use if the material does not fill the allotted time. Some time is needed for "settling in" with each class period. An anecdote connecting the teacher or learner to the subject matter is a nice transition from the real world to the artificial world of the classroom. Some tips that may help the lecture are:

- Put a brief outline of the material to be presented on the blackboard.
- Break the group into smaller groups to discuss particular problems.
- Use demonstrations or movies to break up a lecture.
- Summarize the main points at the end of the lecture. (Mc-Keachie, 1978, p. 23)

Delivery is important, that is, using variation in vocal pitch and volume, looking at the audience, and omitting stereotyped, distracting behaviors. A good lecture arouses an attitude of expectancy in students. Use of clinical data and concrete examples helps students discover their own solutions. An example of outstanding patient management by a nurse practitioner reinforces the content and also carries the message that "You, too, can be a competent, creative provider of care."

Cost/benefit

The lecture method is cost effective especially if the lectures are to be repeated and initial preparation is not excessive. However, it is not cost effective if the lecture repeats content assigned in textbooks and journals. Large numbers can be taught, but other means, such as discussion, must be used to validate learning and get feedback about the effectiveness of the lecture.

In summary, the advantages of the lecture method are:

- Large numbers can hear a lecture.
- They can be repeated with minimal preparation.
- Students and teachers are familiar and comfortable with this method.
- The teacher can organize, present, and interpret recent developments in the content area.

The principle disadvantages are:

- A degree of performing skill is needed; therefore, lectures are deadly if delivery is poor, regardless of the content.
- Students can become preoccupied with notetaking.
- Some additional method is needed to assure student feedback.
- The first presentation requires considerable preparation.

Tips for use in primary care

In lecturing for primary care as in any applied content, the two primary aims are to make the class meaningful to all levels of students and to present information so that the application to clinical practice is apparent. To meet the first goal, it is necessary to know the students' level of knowledge before the class is given. A discussion or pretest can accomplish this so that gaps in knowledge of essential content can be identified and remedied. Most students need a review of relevant anatomy and often physiology concepts also. Most lecture content is aimed at the middle range of student capabilities, but by providing examples of varying difficulty, all students can extend their knowledge of the subject matter.

As noted earlier, lectures are best used to integrate and clarify concepts by giving examples of their application. One example is in teaching epidemiological principles. After an initial reading assignment, a lecture can be used to give multiple examples in the use of the principles. In a pediatric program, examples could be given related to screening of school children. A gerontological program might emphasize identification of chronic diseases. Unusual examples help students understand the application of a concept. For example, using epidemiology to identify patients with mental health problems may help imbed the knowledge more than the usual applications to infectious diseases.

Some form of interchange between students and teacher will indicate the range of understanding. Discussion of examples allows students to demonstrate whether they are able to apply and synthesize content. The ultimate test, of course, is application in clinical practice.

GROUP DISCUSSION

Group discussion is useful in accomplishing many of the aims for which the lecture method is weakest. Discussions can be used to consolidate knowledge already acquired through other methods rather than to impart factual knowledge. Discussion also seems to clarify information and provoke further thought and study. The level of student involvement is raised by establishing rapport, providing feedback about progress, and helping develop skills in formulating and expressing ideas and opinions. By hearing other students' questions and answers, additional impromptu learning takes place. Group process can also be analyzed following the discussion period.

Discussion is a mainstay of any teaching-learning activity and can be used interspersed in a lecture, used with a panel of experts, and elicited through student or teacher leadership. The discussion format and preparatory assignments should be made known in advance.

Skills needed

To have a successful discussion, both time and organization are required. Students resent a lecture disguised as a discussion period; they also resent an unfocused discussion where they are subjected to biased and unsubstantiated opinions from peers.

As in the lecture method, the teachers' knowledge and personality affect success. The teacher can serve in one or more roles in a discussion: as expert, facilitator, or perhaps a socializing agent. As a facilitator some preplanning is necessary. Although the discussion is usually led by the teacher, students (especially graduate students) can assume the leadership role. Nurse educators writing about discussion techniques noted eleven behaviors used by teachers that they labeled discussion-stoppers (Eaton, Davis, & Benner, 1977). [The first six were originally identified by Napell (1976)].

1. *Insufficient waiting time* after an initial question. Complex responses require thinking time. Many teachers can't tolerate a period of silence while students formulate answers. This discourages thoughtful responses.

2. *The rapid reward.* Rapid approval quickly discourages further extension of the idea by other students. Indiscriminate reward, that is, continuously nodding, smiling, and verbal approval is not as effective as judiciously used approval.
3. *The programmed answer.* These are the dead-end questions that elicit a "yes"or "no" type answer rather than encourage application or expansion of knowledge. These do not invite thoughtful responses. Some questions such as, "Do you think taking a more complete history might have helped reach a correct diagnosis?" confirms the teacher's thought processes without helping the student broaden understanding.
4. *Nonspecific feedback question.* Asking if students understand an explanation gets meaningless responses. Few students will admit to not comprehending what a teacher says. Requesting an example which applies the content under discussion will evaluate learning better than a global request for feedback.
5. *Teacher's ego-stroking.* If the teacher becomes the ultimate authority and dominates the discussion, students will not risk making a mistake. For example, after allowing extended comment about a patient problem, the teacher says, "When you have practiced as long as I have, you'll know that . . ." Threatening with a tough grading policy is another form of teacher ego-stroking.
6. *Fixation at a low level of question.* Many teachers ask only questions that require simple recall. Discussions are more profitably used for application, analysis, synthesis, or evaluation. Presenting relevant problems that are challenging, demand creativity, or lead to new approaches helps students to a higher level of cognitive understanding. For example, after a discussion of the management of adult-onset diabetes, a patient problem could be presented where concurrent financial difficulties are a constraint on patient compliance. This also helps resynthesize traditional nursing care into a primary care context.
7. *Intrusive questioning.* Pursuing a student's personal feelings or experience to the point of embarrassment or retreat turns the student off and sometimes the group as well. Both verbal and nonverbal cues must be monitored carefully to avoid going too far. A student who has a health problem herself or in her family

may willingly share the experience while others find such a request intrusive.

8. *Judgmental response to student responses.* Students and teachers often reflect their own cultural or religious bias. Stereotyped generalizations by the teacher about characteristics of groups, whether students or patients, reveal the teacher's biases and prejudices and add little to the students' understanding of the content. Controversial topics such as child care practices, abortion, and prolongation of life tend to elicit strong opinions which must be acknowledged. If, in the teacher's judgment, a student's opinions will be a hindrance to practice, a private conference should be scheduled to explore the problem.

9. *Cutting students off.* Putting students' questions off to a later time discourages further interest and participation. This happens often at the end of a class when the teacher states that there is only time for "burning" questions. If students wander from the topic, refocusing techniques such as summarizing and redirecting are more profitable than cutting students off sharply. Nonverbal teacher behavior such as clock-watching is as effective at stopping discussion as are verbal cut-offs.

10. *Creating a powerful emotional atmosphere and then ignoring feelings.* Once an emotionally-charged response is given, the teacher must deal with it, even though it may have been elicited inadvertently. An example is a student who has a family member who died through improper treatment of the illness under discussion. The teacher must respond to both the feeling and the content of the response.

Eble (1976) suggests that the teacher as discussion leader needs to ask real, not canned questions, have enthusiasm, if not approval, for all responses, and to develop a rhythm in asking a series of questions.

One of the more formal discussion techniques is the *Socratic method*. It has a long history in education, particularly in law and medicine, but few teachers take time to learn the essentials of its use. Socrates believed that there was no teaching, only recollecting. Accordingly, the answers to a problem must lie innately within the individual and can be elicited by judicious and persistent questioning. The method is used and misused by teachers in health-related education with little knowledge of its fundamentals. Actually, the frequent need to solve problems in practice makes the Socratic method valuable when properly used. Essentially, the student is led through defining the problem and examining one or more solutions by rationally testing the alternatives. At the core of Socratic questioning is the discomfort of the respondent who struggles to recall pertinent knowledge. The original intent of this affective reaction was as a motivation to further inquiry; however, this discomfort can degenerate into the humiliation and devastation of the student. This reaction paralyzes rather than motivates. (The teacher who elicits such responses is reminded that such student reaction led to Socrates' death!) Tension can be reduced through keeping the dialogue short, shifting questions to another student, using humor, and clarifying the previous discussion through reexamination of the facts or issues.

The Socratic method, properly used, is appropriate with complex issues of diagnosis and management where the "answer" seems obvious at first. A typical example is a patient suffering from asthma and hypertension where the drug therapy for one may exacerbate the other. Interaction of personal and family problems is another.

The Socratic method is probably more effective with more advanced students because they have a secure knowledge base and self-concept. It is most effective when there is not a tight time schedule so that replies are thoughtful. However, the method can be used judiciously in clinical situations to help a student focus and recall knowledge about a particular problem.

Teachers who use the Socratic method, or who believe they do, would do well to examine its history, assumptions, and classic uses. Hyman (1970, pp. 58–82) presents a good review.

Cost/benefit

The principal direct cost of the discussion method of teaching is in the time teachers and students use to prepare in advance. A more commonly experienced cost is the wasting of time during discussion through nonpreparation or through some of the negative techniques mentioned earlier. The benefits of discussion are increased student understanding of complex ideas and the opportunity to learn from peers.

Tips for use in primary care

Application of content about patient diagnosis and management is an ideal use of discussion whether Socratic or in a less directed way. Discussion of actual cases later in class promotes understanding of fine points not possible in the limited time in the clinical setting. By using recent examples from students' own experiences, several modes of learning are used. The memory of a clinical situation will serve as the prototype for learning the management of a specific problem much better than rote memorization from books. Discussion time will be more productive if the details of the problem can be circulated earlier so that there is time for library research. A situation or problem may be presented through use of audiovisual means or by simulation.

If the discussion is on controversial issues such as third party reimbursement or a new treatment modality, it is helpful to present a summary of the various points of view so that all students have the information. In a discussion with definite pros and cons these can be listed on a blackboard throughout the discussion. A guest speaker or panel where the members have divergent views can serve to crystallize the issues. For instance, a discussion of the roles of health team members can be initiated by a panel made up of members of an existing team. They can be asked to discuss not only the advantages of health team membership but also some of the problems.

In summary, discussion can clarify concepts and other cognitive knowledge and stimulate students to study further on their own. Students and teachers need to prepare for discussion through reading or watching media presentations. The affective tone of a discussion group needs attention as well as the subject matter. Nurse practitioners and others in expanded roles profit from discussion concerning complex management problems as well as role-oriented issues.

SEMINARS

The seminar is a special form of the discussion method used primarily in upper division or graduate education. Originally, the term denoted a small group of students engaged in advanced study and research under the aegis of a faculty member. Realistically, it has come to mean a small discussion group, perhaps twenty students or less. As in larger discussion groups, seminars presuppose that students come with a certain amount of knowledge on the given topic. The culminating activity of a seminar is often an issue-oriented paper. Small work groups can be formed to develop topics of common interest. The topics can be patient-centered or role issues.

The teacher's role in the seminar can be the same as in any discussion group. In addition, the drawing out of students' knowledge and experience on the seminar topic assumes greater importance at a graduate or continuing education level. Many students have extensive experience that could be helpful to themselves or their peers yet they are reticent to share it. Sensitivity and skill in eliciting contributions will enhance the seminar for all.

In the seminar, more than in other groups, students may serve as leaders. The teacher, then, has an additional task—to train students in discussion leading.

Seminars are appropriate in graduate and continuing education programs in primary care, particularly for complex issues. Some of these issues are delineated in Chapter 2. Legal issues are a good topic for seminars because students come with a variety of concerns and need for knowledge. Material can be presented and discussed that meets individual needs. Ethical dilemmas facing nurse practitioners, legislative issues, and private practice are vital concerns that adapt well to the seminar format. It is also an appropriate method for discussion of new approaches to patient care or newly recognized health problems, such as Reye's syndrome in children, alternate birthing centers in women's health, or AIDS.

AUDIOVISUAL MEDIA

Media laboratories are now a standard resource in most hospitals and schools of nursing. The equipment (projectors, recorders, etc.) to use most forms of media are also readily available to nursing instruction. Media can be used in the classroom interspersed throughout a lecture or discussion, for independent learning, and for clinical conferences. Properly used audiovisual materials can: (1) increase understanding of a topic; (2) add interest to a subject; (3) teach a skill; (4) demonstrate and promote positive attitudes; and (5) offer experiences not easily obtained elsewhere (Kemp, 1963). Additionally, audiovisual aids can stimulate and provoke further investigation by the student, allow for remedial work, or challenge a gifted student.

To further cognitive learning, still pictures such as overheads or slides can be used during a class to present an outline of topics and emphasize important concepts and key words. Research studies with statistics are better understood when charts and graphs supplement verbal presentation. Moving pictures (movies, videotapes) of clinical interviews, human behavior, or case presentations are excellent for promoting problem solving or application, synthesis, and evaluation of content already addressed. Some examples of use of media in a nurse practitioner program are given below.

- *Example 1:* The use of a video or audio taped interview of a patient with the problem being discussed. Students can then be asked to identify additional data needed and/or give a tentative diagnosis and plan.
- *Example 2:* Two different patient provider interactions to compare and contrast interview techniques.
- *Example 3:* Slides to demonstrate normal gross or microscopic anatomy or pathological findings.

A common use of audiovisual aids in expanded programs is the demonstration of psychomotor skills, the physical examination in particular. Several series for both adults' and children's exams are available commercially or a skilled examiner can be filmed. Developmental testing such as the Brazelton Neonatal Assessment Scale or the Bayley Scales of Infant Development is illustrated best by moving pictures or video. These have the advantage of being able to show change over time, something a live demonstration cannot do efficiently. Similarly, the progress of a woman through pregnancy, labor, and delivery can be demonstrated through moving pictures or a series of illustrations made into slides.

Affective learning can also be facilitated with audiovisual media. Attitude formation is enhanced by showing interaction of patients or colleagues role-played or recorded in life. Ethical and moral issues are sometimes the subject of commercial programs such as "All In The Family."

Each form of media has uses and limitations that are summarized in Table 7-1.

Choosing the best medium

New instructors are bewildered by the many types of software available for the health professions. The use of audiovisual aids requires planning that should begin as soon as the content is determined. Time is needed to order, ship, and preview media.

A recently available method of identifying what is available for a given topic is the AVLINE computerized search through the National Library of Medicine (Bridgman & Suter, 1979). Titles and descriptions of audiovisual instructional materials can be accessed by using the same medical subject headings and computer access as used for a MEDLINE literature search (Medical Subject Headings, 1984). The search can be narrowed further by specifying certain types of equipment. Materials are designated as self-instructional or lecture support. The search can provide abstracts from which the teacher determines its suitability. The name of the producer is included with an address and phone number so that units can be ordered for preview.

Other methods can be used to find appropriate modules. Any institution that has a media laboratory or learning resource center should have catalogs from various media distributors. In addition, medical, social work, or other behavior and biological science departments have media libraries from which nursing faculty can borrow. Obviously, much time can be wasted in tracking down resources. New teachers should be oriented to resources in their setting.

Presentation of visual media

Choosing the proper module is the first step. Improper display or projection is irritating and disappointing to students and may leave a negative attitude about the content. Some principles for use of

Table 7-1.   Uses of Audiovisual Media

	Objects	Still Pictures
Cognitive Learning	Useful with demonstrations. Use to teach recognition, principles, sequential steps, rules. Can see, feel, and manipulate real objects. Not useful in large groups.	Useful in small groups or for individuals. Use to present sequences, teach concepts, recognition, give visual cues.
Psycho-motor Learning	Real objects useful for practice in skills, i.e., computers, stethoscope. Models useful in teaching configuration, i.e., anatomy. Use people to demonstrate actions.	Little use except to show relative positions, i.e., anatomical chart, while practicing skills.
Affective Learning	Limited application except to use objects as focus of desired attitude. Real people showing emotions or expressing feelings can be useful with discussion and reading.	Limited application. Can use with audio to influence attitudes.
	Audio	Moving Pictures or Video
Cognitive Learning	Use with any size group. Useful for monitoring student-patient interaction. Best used with printed or projected media. Requires little training to produce if high quality not required.	Use with any size group. Useful for teaching processes, events, ideas, to dramatize content. Holds attention. Recreates patient encounters. Can be created with portable equipment and some training.

Table 7-1.   Uses of Audiovisual Media (continued)

Psycho-Motor Learning	Useful only when demonstrating speech or hearing-related skills, i.e., breath sounds. Useful with objects or slides.	Very useful to model skills, demonstrate processes over time, give feedback on student-patient encounters. Can be used for testing and evaluation. Useful for recording events or physical behaviors.
Affective Learning	Limited application. May be used to establish moods, i.e., background music or narration. In group work, may be used to play back discussion and focus attitudes. Use with slides for greater impact.	Very useful for influencing attitudes. Drama or real life playback. Excellent for triggering discussion on values.

nonprojected materials (photographic prints, drawings, illustrations, real objects, models, chalk boards) are:

- Illustrate only one major idea or principle with each unit.
- Illustrations should be large enough for all to see—don't use nonprojected illustrations in front of a large group.
- Display or mount materials.

- Point out what area of the picture, model, or object is being discussed.
- Make the materials available for careful viewing after teaching.

Projected material (slides, motion pictures, overhead or opaque projections, filmstrips, videotapes) also are more effective when used properly. Suggested steps are:

1. Preview the material and take notes to use while teaching.
2. Use an evaluation form to keep on file after the first use.
3. Have the room and equipment ready in advance. Check technical aspects of focus and sound.
4. Discuss with students what they will see before showing, to structure the experience and create interest.
5. Stop the presentation for discussion, if necessary.
6. Follow up with appropriate activities such as discussion, practice of a skill, or assignment (Davis & Schenk, 1978).

Cost/benefit

If a program is well funded, a library of audiovisual materials can be acquired over time. If there is no budget for purchase of units, many can be borrowed for little or no charge. Occasionally drug companies loan materials on disease processes or management. Manufacturers of equipment have "how-to-use" audiovisual units. Although the initial cost may be high, audiovisual units can save in other areas such as hiring of experts to teach complex material.

Production of units by individual teachers or programs is possible. Generally, it is not cost effective if a commercial unit is available that covers the needed content. Production of commercial quality units requires much time from nursing and media experts. Kemp (1963) offers guidelines for planning and producing audiovisual materials.

TEAM TEACHING

Because nurses preparing for an expanded role need to integrate content from several disciplines, team teaching is an appropriate technique. However, in examining the advantages and disadvantages in the nursing literature many precautions appear.

The first problem is to define what is meant by team teaching. The purest form is the participation of all faculty assigned to a course in planning, teaching, and evaluating. Classroom teaching then is done by the faculty member who has the most expertise in the content area. This may mean coteaching a particular class or dividing up the classes among team members. All teachers attend all classes and contribute their expertise to the discussion.

It is readily apparent that the major disadvantage to team teaching is the time involved for several teachers. In an interdisciplinary course such as one requiring the expertise of medical and other specialities, it is unrealistic for all team members to attend all classes. Perhaps the most one can hope for is participation of all pertinent disciplines in the planning and evaluation phases. Then individual teachers from each discipline can be responsible for individual classes.

Even in courses involving only nursing faculty, the team concept can degenerate after the first implementation. Hogstel and Ackley (1979) noted that, in an integrated baccalaureate curriculum, the instructors who were not teaching a class often corrected papers or read during classes. This author has noted similar distracting behavior including whispering and passing of notes between teachers, a severe form of negative role-modeling. On the other hand, if the team is not required to attend all classes, individual teacher responsibility seems to suffer. When students ask for information, the team member may say that since she or he didn't teach that content they can't help the student. Students are confused and, additionally, denied the different points of view from specialists.

In an expanded-role nursing program, if true interdisciplinary teaching is not possible, the curriculum content and its implementation should be controlled by nursing. In essence, the course is then coordinated by a nursing instructor who is responsible for the orientation of other teachers. Thus, some distinction needs to be made between team members who have overall responsibility and others who are brought in as guest lecturers. Those in the latter category should be given the objectives for the class and offered help in translating them into class content. The nursing coordinator attends and is responsible for evaluation of students in the content area. Often guest lecturers miss the mark because they do not have the necessary information to prepare the classes. Students then see the input of other specialists as irrelevant or too esoteric. Team teaching can be enhanced by adhering to the following guidelines:

1. Have regular team meetings.
2. Encourage discussion of problems and approaches.
3. Share responsibility for quality teaching among all team members.
4. Develop course and class objectives mutually.
5. Set up ground rules for team participation during classes.
6. Orient new faculty to the process of team teaching.
7. Explain the team approach to students.
8. Include teaching methods in the course evaluation. (Hogstel and Ackley, 1979, pp. 50–51).

ASSIGNMENTS

Students may fail to consider assignments as instructional modes, but that is their basic goal. The purposes of out-of-classroom assignments are to:

1. Further clarify the content or concept taught.
2. Reinforce new learning.
3. Enhance transfer of learning to a broader class of situations.
4. Give practice in problem solving.
5. Actively involve the learner.
6. Provide opportunities to apply learning to clinical problems.
7. Present several views on a controversial subject.
8. Meet individual learning needs.

Assignments may be given before or after content is presented in class. The learning style of a particular student or group may determine which is more effective. Essential content is best assigned before a lecture and application exercises after. Some traditional assignments are discussed below while less traditional modes are covered in Chapter 9.

Textbooks

Choosing of texts for an expanded-role course is problematic. Comprehensive medical texts are expensive and treat psychosocial implications lightly, if at all. Few nursing texts include diagnosis and management in enough depth to be used alone. Several texts have been prepared by or for nurse practitioners in primary care, but none are comprehensive enough to be used alone. How many books students are required to purchase depends on the availability and adequacy of library facilities. If books can be put on reserve and reliably available, fewer need to be purchased.

Assignments in texts should be of reasonable length and not duplicative. Before making reading assignments the teacher should ask, "What new information does this reading add?" It is most helpful to have suggested readings as well as required ones for the highly motivated student or for those who need many different sources for learning. Indicating readings for prerequisite knowledge such as anatomy, physiology, or pathology allows students to supplement their background knowledge independently.

Papers

Papers assigned in an expanded-role course are not usually an exercise in creative writing, but are expository in nature. Early papers can be used to assess writing and research skills. Issue-oriented topics force students to read, analyze, and present different viewpoints. An emphasis on recognizing and controlling the student's bias has applications in later courses on patient management.

Papers that are at the application, synthesis, or evaluation level are more effective than those asking only for a compilation of facts. The purpose and evaluation criteria for each paper should be clearly delineated at the time the assignment is made. A general outline is helpful for the purpose. Some students, particularly those in a continuing education program, need an introduction to obtaining resources. Cooperative librarians can help compile a list of commonly used sources in nursing. Orientation to the many computerized literature searches expands the tools available for independent learning.

Programmed instruction

Computer-assisted learning and printed programs and texts are forms of programmed instruction. The advantages of this mode are in its structure, the immediate feedback, and the self-study characteristics. Learning is divided into very small, incremental steps.

Disadvantages of programmed instruction are the need to find or develop the desired program, obtain the equipment or books, and instruct students in their use. Specific cognitive knowledge is appropriately presented through programmed learning but may take more study time than reading texts. Nevertheless, the additional involvement of the learner may negate these disadvantages. Some students enjoy the logical pace of programmed learning, but others who learn in intuitive leaps find it tedious.

The cost of purchasing programs or computer access may be prohibitive. However, if the course is based at a large university, medical teaching facility, or large hospital, programmed learning books or computer terminals may already be available. Many of the computer-assisted programs developed for medical students and physicians can be used in conjunction with nursing content.

Case studies

Case studies are disguised under many names such as patient problems or record audits. The goal is to analyze a data base and/or plan for a patient's care at various stages of diagnosis or management. Cases are used best following presentation of didactic material to promote generalization of knowledge. One method is to distribute what amounts to a complete case history. The student's task is to formulate a diagnosis and plan, either orally or in writing. Group discussion after completion of the assignment should provide several different approaches that can be evaluated.

A refinement of this technique is the distribution of an incomplete subjective, objective, assessment, and plan (SOAP) with data missing. The student must first recognize what additional data are needed, then formulate the assessment and plan. Some computer programs are variations of this theme and give feedback not only on correctness of the answers but also on the efficiency of obtaining them.

In most case studies, the teacher must be ready to acknowledge unusual but equally correct responses given by some students. This is an opportunity to consider together the probability of a diagnosis being correct or the proposed plan being effective. In fact, such experiences reinforce the existence of much ambiguity found in "real-world" patient management.

In summary, many techniques are available to enhance student learning. No one method is best for all content and all students. Table 7-2 lists most of the commonly used teaching methods and the goals for each.

Primary care nursing is practice-oriented; therefore, methods should be chosen that promote generalization of didactic content to clinical practice. Techniques that actively involve and motivate the learner are more useful than passive spoon-feeding by the teacher. Moreover, promoting independence and development of the student's own resources encourages professional learning throughout a career.

HELPING STUDENTS LEARN

Instructional methods can be appropriately chosen and sleekly executed, yet students may not learn or—even more devastating to the teacher—may not be motivated to learn. What goes wrong? Individual student learning and motivation can be vexing to a conscientious instructor. The relatively new fields of adult learning and development theory shed some light on how professional students, presumably adults, may be helped. The theory of androgogy is attractive in its rational approach substantiated by knowledge of adult development. Androgogy, the teaching of adults, as opposed to pedagogy, the teaching of children, is based on four assumptions derived from knowledge of adult development (Knowles, 1978).

1. *As a person grows and matures, the self-concept moves from total dependency to increased self-directedness.* Androgogy as-

Table 7-2. Checklist of Teaching Techniques

TECHNIQUE	GOALS POTENTIALLY ACHIEVED
Books	Knowledge Critical thinking
Lecture	Knowledge Inspiration, motivations (a "cutting edge" lecture) Identification by a scholar Critical thinking (by example)
Discussion	Critical thinking Relating knowledge to student experiences Application Attitude change
Modular Instruction	Knowledge, application, and other (depends upon type of tests and tutoring)
Student panel, student reports	Interest and motivation (at least for participants)
Guest lecturer or resource person	Added interest and information
Films	Makes material more concrete Facilitates learning materials involving motion or visual detail Interest

TV	Interest (greater involvement than film)
	Motion, visual details
Slides	Permit visual materials to be greatly enlarged and held in view while explained
	Interest
Bulletin boards, mock-up	Provide opportunity for learning at student's own pace
	May help student relate learning in classrooms to materials presented in mass media
	Provide concrete examples
Recordings	Provide concrete auditory experience
	Taped recordings can be made cheaply by instructor to bring situations outside the classroom to the class
Field trips	First-hand knowledge
	Interest
Laboratory	First-hand experience
	Scientific method
Role playing	Real-life experience
	Develops human relations skills
	Interest
Buzz groups	Create awareness of problems
	Practice in problem solving
	Increased involvement

Table 7-2. *(continued)*

TECHNIQUE	GOALS POTENTIALLY ACHIEVED
Study guides, workbooks	Aid organization and learning of materials Promote application of knowledge
Periodicals	Bridge gap between classroom and other experience of students
Teaching machines and programmed texts	Learning knowledge and skills, particularly those requiring repetition and immediate feedback
Computer-aided instruction	Potentially can achieve any of these goals when combined with other materials, but currently limited by availability of college-level programs

Used by permission from W. J. McKeachie. Teaching Tips: A Guide for the Beginning College Teacher, 7th edition, 1978. Lexington, Massachusetts: D. C. Heath and Company, pp. 296-297.

sumes that an individual is psychologically an adult when he achieves a self-concept of essential self-direction. Knowles points out that students who have entered professional school or a job are identifying as an adult and that any experience they perceive as being treated as children decreases learning.

2. *With maturity, an individual has an expanding reservoir of experience that is a rich resource for learning.* New learnings can be related to this broadening base. Accordingly, there should be an emphasis on experiental techniques such as discussion, laboratory, simulation, field experiences rather than more passive techniques such as lectures, media presentations, and assigned readings. Knowles adds that an adult's experience is part of identity. If previous experience is devalued or ignored, students perceive it as a rejection of a part of their personal identity.

3. *With maturity, readiness to learn is based more on developmental tasks and needs of roles than on biological development or academic pressure.* The implication is that learning experiences must coincide with the learner's developmental tasks. This translates into providing experiences from which the student may learn or helping the student learn from past experiences.

4. *Adults' orientation to learning is based on the need to cope with perceived life problems.* On the contrary, children learn to get to the next academic step rather than learning for the immediate application of knowledge. Adults learn what they believe can be applied in the near future and are primarily problem-oriented.

Readers who teach registered nurses in continuing education or graduate programs may find that the theory of androgogy provides insight into problems they have experienced. For example, one student in a master's program to prepare nurse practitioners appeared at an appointment with her advisor very upset. Although she had done well the previous semester, she felt unprepared and inadequate after a few days of clinical experience as a primary health care provider. More crushing was the fact that she had received a low "C" on the first test in clinical problems. With minimal direction from her advisor, she was able to discern that her work load and schedule must be changed to provide more study time. In this case, her positive self-concept as a good student and as a self-directed adult were helpful.

Students often complain that classes are "disconnected" or "not relevant." Whereas children will learn because the teacher says it is important, adults need to know that content will be applicable to their need. If not all students see these connections with real-life problems, the teacher can provide bridges from their previous experience or provide clinical examples.

Accepting the theory of androgogy does not mean that older theories, for example, conditioning or field theories, do not apply. It merely offers another way to view the adult learner. Knowles sees the teacher as a facilitator of learning rather than a "teller" of knowledge. He cites and supports Rogers' often-quoted observation that "teaching . . . is a vastly overrated function" (Rogers, 1969, p. 103). In Table 7-3 some principles of teaching are listed based on androgogical theory.

How can these principles be used in teaching expanded-role students who must reach a certain level of competence for safe practice? Although the instructor knows what a nurse practitioner, nurse midwife, or other nurse in an expanded role needs to know to practice competently, it will be more effective for the student to discover this through experience. Observation of another nurse practitioner or direct patient care will help the student set objectives that are congruent with role requirements and to evaluate performance by these standards. The teacher can help students organize their own learning and suggest techniques to meet their needs.

The teacher serves as a role model with three possible effects (Bandura and Walters, 1963):

- modeling effect to acquire new responses
- inhibit or disinhibit previously acquired responses
- cues are received to release responses that are neither new nor inhibited.

Teachers in a practice profession are models to students whether or not this is consciously acknowledged. This effect is even more important in expanded roles where students may have little previous contact with potential role models prior to entering the program. They may tend to model physicians they know or nurses in more

Table 7-3. Role of the Teacher in Androgogical Teaching

CONDITIONS OF LEARNING	PRINCIPLES OF TEACHING
The learners feel a need to learn.	1. The teacher exposes students to new possibilities of self-fulfillment. 2. The teacher helps each student clarify his own aspirations for improved behavior. 3. The teacher helps each student diagnose the gap between his aspirations and his present level of performance. 4. The teacher helps the students identify the life problems they experience because of the gaps in their personal equipment.
The learning environment is characterized by physical comfort, mutual trust and respect, mutual helpfulness, freedom of expression, and acceptance of differences.	5. The teacher provides physical conditions that are comfortable (as to seating, smoking, temperature, ventilation, lighting, decoration) and conducive to interaction (preferably, no person sitting behind another person). 6. The teacher accepts each student as a person of worth and respects his feelings and ideas. 7. The teacher seeks to build relationships of mutual trust and helpfulness among students by encouraging cooperative activities and refraining from inducing competitiveness and judgmentalness. 8. The teacher exposes his own feelings and contributes his resources as a colearner in the spirit of mutual inquiry.
The learners perceive the goals of a learning experience to be their goals.	9. The teacher involves the students in a mutual process of formulating learning objectives in which the needs of the students, of the institution, and of the society are taken into account.

Table 7-3. (*continued*)

CONDITIONS OF LEARNING	PRINCIPLES OF TEACHING
The learners accept a share of the responsibility for planning and operating a learning experience, and therefore have a feeling of commitment toward it.	10. The teacher shares his thinking about options available in the designing of learning experiences and the selection of materials and methods and involves the students in deciding among these options jointly. 11. The teacher helps the students to organize themselves (project groups, learning-teaching teams, independent study, etc.) to share responsibility in the process of mutual inquiry.
The learners participate actively in the learning process.	12. The teacher helps the students exploit their own experiences as resources for learning through the use of such techniques as discussion, role playing, case method, etc.
The learning process is related to and makes use of the experience of the learners.	13. The teacher gears the presentation of his own resources to the levels of experience of his particular students. 14. The teacher helps the students apply new learning to their experience, and thus to make the learnings more meaningful and integrated.
The learners have a sense of progress toward their goals.	15. The teacher involves the students in developing mutually acceptable criteria and methods for measuring progress toward the learning objectives. 16. The teacher helps the students develop and apply procedures for self-evaluation according to these criteria.

From <u>The Adult Learner: A Neglected Species,</u> 2nd ed., by Malcolm Knowles. ©1978 by Gulf Publishing Company, Houston, Texas. All rights reserved. Used with permission.

traditional roles. In trying on new roles students observe their instructor for cues. If the cues are not clear or are inconsistent with student expectations, confusion results. An assignment to observe several nurses in different settings followed by a discussion of the expanded role may be more helpful than only assigned readings.

Sociocultural aspects of learning

If adult students base their learning on previous experience, it is apparent that those who come from a minority ethnic or cultural background will need help in making connections from their experiences to new learning. Language or writing difficulties compound the problem. These students need to perceive that their backgrounds and experience are as valuable as those of the majority. Older or younger students may need help in seeing what they bring of value to the classroom.

SUMMARY

Many instructional methods are available. No one mode is best for all content or, for that matter, all students. A sensitive teacher matches the method to students and content. More importantly, feedback is elicited and used to replan to meet individual as well as group needs.

REFERENCES

Bandura, A. & Walters, R. H. *Social learning and personality development.* New York: Holt, Rinehart and Winston, 1963.

Bloom, B. S. (Ed.). *Taxonomy of educational objectives: Handbook 1: Cognitive Domain.* New York: Longmans, Inc., 1977.

Bridgman, C. F. & Suter, E. Searching AVLINE for curriculum-related audiovisual instructional materials. *Journal of Medical Education*, 1979, 54, 236–237.

Conley, V. C. *Curriculum and instruction in nursing.* Boston: Little, Brown and Company, 1973.

Davis, R. M. & Schenk, B. *Media handbook: A guide to selecting, producing, and using media for patient education programs.* Chicago: American Hospital Association, 1978.

Eaton, S., Davis, G. L., & Benner, P. E. Discussion stoppers in teaching. *Nursing Outlook*, 1977, *25*, 578–583.

Eble, I. E. *The craft of teaching: A guide to mastering the professor's art.* San Francisco: Jossey-Bass, 1976.

Edinberg, M. A., Dodson, S. E., & Veach, T. L. A preliminary study of student learning in interdisciplinary health teams. *Journal of Medical Education*, 1978, *53*, 667–671.

Hogstel, M. O. & Ackley, N. L. Making team teaching work. *Nursing Outlook*, 1979, *27*, 48–51.

Hyman, R. T. *Ways of teaching.* Philadelphia: J. B. Lippincott Company, 1970.

Jason, H. The relevance of medical education to medical practice. *JAMA*, *212*, 2092–2095.

Kemp, J. E. *Planning and producing audiovisual materials.* San Francisco: Chandler Publishing Company, 1963.

Knowles, M. S. *The adult learner: A neglected species*, 2nd ed. Houston: Gulf Publishing Company, 1978.

McKeachie, W. J. *Teaching tips: A guidebook for the beginning college teacher*, 7th ed. Lexington, Massachusetts: D.C. Heath and Company, 1978.

Medical Subject Headings, U.S. Department of Health and Human Services, Public Health Service, National Institute of Health, National Library of Medicine, 1984.

Napell, S. M. Six common nonfacilitating teaching behaviors. *Contemporary Education*, 1976, *47*, 79–82.

Rogers, C. *Freedom to learn: A view of what education might become.* Columbus, Ohio: Charles E. Merrill, Publishing Co., 1969.

8

Clinical Instruction

Careful planning of clinical experience is essential in preparing nurses for expanded roles. Students and teachers perceive success in the clinical arena as the ultimate test of knowledge and skills—and correctly so. An effective nurse practitioner must apply highly complex didactic learning to diverse client situations; being able to recite the information is not enough. The clinical nursing instructor can, by selecting and structuring learning opportunities, facilitate the student's efforts. In this chapter the following topics will be considered:

- faculty preceptors
- sites for clinical teaching
- teaching assessment
- teaching diagnosis and management
- presentation and recording of data
- moving toward independence.

FACULTY PRECEPTORS

Who should teach expanded-role students in the clinical area? More programs now have the luxury of debating this issue as the number of prepared nurse faculty increases. In the early years of the nurse practitioner movement most didactic and clinical teaching was done by physicians. Often nursing faculty learned along with their first class, then assumed more responsibility for clinical teaching as their skills increased.

In spite of increased preparation, most nursing faculty believe that interdisciplinary teaching is essential to prepare for practice in an interdisciplinary health care setting. In addition to the technical knowledge physicians and other clinicians bring, issues such as the overlapping of roles, ownership of the patient, and differing theoretical approaches to practice are more likely to be faced with both nurses and physicians involved. Nursing faculty should be prepared to teach assessment skills (history and physical) alone except in isolated areas where continuing education programs for faculty development are not available. Psychosocial assessment of groups such as families or particular ethnic or cultural groups can be taught by other nurses or specialists with expertise in the needed area. Developmental assessment of children may be in the purview of several disciplines—nursing, medicine, psychology, or child development specialists. Even when teaching specialty assessment content, a guest instructor should be made aware of the nature of the role for which students are being prepared, and the objectives of the content being taught. Although input can be sought from the visiting instructor, content, objectives, and evaluation are best retained by those responsible for the total course.

Precepting of students in clinical sites where teaching diagnosis and management is the purpose is best accomplished through some form of nurse-physician team. The roles and responsibilities of each are worked out based on considerations such as expertise, personality, role in the agency, needs of students, and stage of the course or program. Some of the tasks that may be shared or divided are:

1. Selecting patients.
2. Observing students as they perform assessment skills.
3. Listening to student presentations.
4. Monitoring patients' records after they are seen.
5. Providing for follow-up diagnostic tests.
6. Evaluating students.

SITES FOR CLINICAL TEACHING

Clinical placements are chosen to meet clinical objectives. These must be clearly and specifically stated. When overall course objectives are prepared (Chapter 6), sufficient detail may be lacking to define clinical content. Subobjectives should be written to illustrate further the expected outcomes to faculty, students, and staff of the agency. Many cognitive objectives will be at the application level (Bloom, 1977) or higher. Development of new psychomotor skills is a substantial part of the early clinical phase of a nurse practitioner program. Affective behavior is often demonstrated, discussed, and evaluated in clinical settings even though the content may be formally presented in the classroom. All these needs and objectives must be considered in choosing clinical sites.

The specificity of the content, whether by age group (i.e., pediatrics, gerontology) or by specialty (i.e., women's health, hypertension, health screening) will also determine placement to some extent. It is certainly easier to find appropriate learning experiences for women's health content in an ob-gyn setting, but other places such as college health centers or a general adult setting may provide enough patients for meeting objectives.

Generally, the students will benefit most from settings similar to those for which the program prepares graduates. Most nurse practitioner programs prepare for practice in an ambulatory setting. While it once was relatively easy to arrange student placement in a health department or hospital clinic, these agencies are now crowded with students from many professions. Nurse practitioner students compete for placements not only with medical students but also with physicians' assistants, pharmacy students, social work students, and others. Although learning needs are somewhat different, space limitations and access to patients become major obstacles to meeting the needs of multiple students in one setting. Another factor limiting access to ambulatory settings is a growing concern for consumer protection. Facilities that are not part of a teaching institution, and some that are, look carefully at patient satisfaction and cost effectiveness before accepting students. In return, they may expect some benefits to accrue in money or services. Negotiating ambulatory placements is a complex and important process (Jones, 1983). It behooves faculty to approach agencies prepared with well-defined needs and a list of required resources. Agreement should be reached on:

1. Dates and times of rotation.
2. Faculty supervision.
3. Number of students.
4. Experiences needed (objectives to be met).
5. Physical needs (i.e., conference room, parking, lockers).
6. Agency requirements for students (i.e., malpractice insurance, uniforms, badges).
7. Financial arrangements or services school will provide to agency.

A visit to the site can clarify the needs and responsibilities of faculty, students, and staff. Most agencies require a written agreement which can be extended indefinitely. A placement for a single student in an agency or with a solo physician or nurse practitioner is simpler, but the same process is followed. If the nursing faculty will be present with a group of students, a period of faculty orientation saves time later. Periodic evaluation by the faculty and agency staff should be built into the agreement.

Use of in-patient settings for assessment

There is some value in considering in-patient settings in teaching assessment skills and for demonstration of selected pathology. The beginning student is learning interviewing and psychomotor skills that are not only new and complex but veiled in a mystique. Problems may arise if the student is asked to dispense patient care at the same time. Obtaining an initial data base on hospitalized patients decreases the anxiety and enables the student to concentrate on developing skills and on the organization and presentation of findings to the preceptor. This exercise can be performed as the initial admission work-up for a hospitalized patient but a more common practice is for it to be the partial repetition of specific system assessments. There are some disadvantages in using hospitalized patients for repeating examinations. Knafl (1979) found in a small sample that nurse practitioner students in an initial health assessment course thought that interviewing and examining in-patients who had already been assessed was not a "reality" experience compared to later assignments where actual care was provided. The students felt it was an academic, ivory tower exercise and that they had less control than in a later course where they were the primary providers. The disadvantages of using patients who already have a complete data base must be weighed against the advantages. Patients' rights are also a consideration in that repeating an examination is somewhat of an imposition unless it adds to the data base. On the other hand, some patients enjoy the attention from students.

Other possible sites for students to gain assessment experience of relatively well adults are screening programs in industry, community agencies, military installations, health fairs, college health services, residencies for the elderly, prisons, and migrant camps.

Day care centers for children, schools, well-child clinics, hospital nurseries, and private pediatricians' offices are possible sites for assessment of well children. Developmental assessments may be easier to arrange than physical examinations. Consent of the parent or guardian is necessary and should be arranged through the agency. Opportunities to give some type of service—health screening, counseling on risk factors, nutrition, exercise, and safety—provide a way for students to pay back for student placements and increase the perceived value of the experience to the student.

TEACHING ASSESSMENT

The first phase in most expanded-role programs is the teaching of assessment. The content varies with the population to be served. In programs teaching comprehensive primary care the data base for initial assessment includes a history, physical examination, and laboratory data. A comprehensive pediatric program adds a large developmental and family component as well as the mother's labor and delivery history. Specialized programs (i.e., emergency, women's health, and college health) may teach a comprehensive assessment but emphasize the episodic visit.

Approach

The process of obtaining a data base (history, physical, and laboratory data) is most often taught using the medical systems model because of the need to communicate both orally and in writing to physicians and other health team members. This format, however, is often inadequate to reflect the nursing needs of patients. Additions, usually psychosocial data, to the usual medical format through use of a nursing history can round out the data base. These additions should evolve in a systematic way and be consistent with the program's philosophy and conceptual framework. The goal is to teach the process of obtaining a data base for both health and illness care, and not a pieced-together product with overlapping content.

The clinical laboratory

Although assessment may be taught using actual patients, initial demonstration and practice in a skills laboratory is the most effective and efficient approach. Both history taking and physical assessment skills improve following practice on fellow students or with simulated patients. Audiovisual software on these skills are available from several sources. In choosing one or more units for purchase the instructor should consider not only the quality of the product but the message it will convey to the student. Units produced by and for physicians and medical students do little to dispel the student's fear of performing physical examinations. The history taking may also be lacking in psychosocial or health promotion and prevention content, all of major concern to the nurse. On the other hand, units produced for medical students may have more detail, particularly in the identification of abnormal findings, than those produced for nurses. Most companies will allow previews of units before purchase. Those films that also demonstrate history taking as well as physical assessment for the particular system are the best buy.

It is also possible to produce audiovisual units, but it is not cost effective in light of the many commercial products now available. The best use of audio and videotaping resources is for the purpose of critiquing individual interactions rather than presenting the normative content. See Chapter 9 for creative uses of audiovisual software in clinical teaching.

Interviewing and interpersonal skills

History taking or interviewing is a skill nurses are assumed to have, but the open-ended, reflective, nondirected methods most nurses use must be shaped and sharpened to obtain a complete data base efficiently. Sparks, Vitalo, Cohen, and Kahn (1980) surveyed expanded role programs to determine the extent of teaching and evaluation of interpersonal skills and found that 78 percent of the programs included specific content. The majority of programs taught (1) interpersonal process skills; (2) information gathering skills; (3) information giving/counseling skills; and (4) psychosocial intervention skills. It is evident that most programs do not assume that nurses enter an expanded-role program with the interpersonal skills necessary for the expanded role. Other areas in which the researchers found specific content taught were in team membership skills, group problem solving, supervising skills, and interpersonal skills for the physical examination. The necessity to include content and practice in all these areas depends on students' entering skills level and the inclusion of this content elsewhere in the curriculum. For instance, counseling and patient teaching is more appropriately taught under patient management. Certainly interpersonal skills contribute substantially to success in peer and health team contacts as well as with patients.

The techniques for teaching interpersonal skills will vary with the purpose and resources available. The most common content taught in expanded role curricula, that of history taking or information gathering, can first be demonstrated with videotapes, audiotapes, or role playing by instructors. Cultural differences in language and values between nurse practitioner and patients should be emphasized as well as the importance of nonverbal behavior of both parties. Student discomfort with certain aspects of the history (i.e., sexual, financial) may be eased with additional practice in role playing in the clinical laboratory. Several references are listed under suggested readings at the end of the chapter in teaching interviewing and interpersonal skills with patients. The greatest difference in the teaching of interviewing to obtain a data base versus a nondirective approach is the need to guide the interaction without neglecting the patient's (or parents') immediate needs for information or assurance. In essence, history taking is not primarily a therapeutic event but a data-gathering process. Through review of audio or videotapes of student-patient interviews, the instructor can point out where the direction of the conversation might have been guided to obtain better data in a shorter time. As the student progresses, a time limit for obtaining the history is helpful.

INTERVIEWING ACTUAL PATIENTS

Progression from the interviewing of classmates, instructors, or simulated patients should be gradual. The transition is easier if the first "real" patient contacts (1) are not under a severe time constraint; (2) are similar to the student culturally and socially; (3) have no language or other communication barrier; and (4) are not acutely ill.

Experience in obtaining both complete and episodic histories is essential. The decision as to what areas to consider in an episodic visit requires much practice and is an important step in developing clinical judgment. Interviewing of actual clients can be combined with practice of related parts of the physical examination, but the anxiety inherent in practicing new psychomotor skills detracts from developing interviewing skills. Pediatric practitioners need to develop skills in interviewing parents of varying ability to communicate as well as in techniques for interviewing older children and adolescents.

It may be possible to find relatively well patients for interviewing in some ambulatory settings such as industrial clinics or day care centers for senior citizens. However, the reality may be that physical examinations and some management of problems will need to be combined. In this event, even more practice in laboratory situations is necessary to avoid feelings of inadequacy.

The physical examination

Predictably, the learning of physical assessment skills takes on inordinate importance to the new nurse practitioner student. Faced with the use of strange equipment and the learning of skills previously off limits to nurses, the student may experience a level of anxiety akin to that some people feel in learning mathematics or driving a car. Some low to moderate levels of anxiety enhance learning but high levels inhibit it. A thorough and complete orientation and delineation of the expected level of performance are necessary. The parts of the examination that are the most technically difficult for most students are the eye, ear, cardiac, and neurological assessments. Genital examinations are difficult for some. If a student has extensive experience in some specialties, this is helpful to her and to classmates. Students are unexpected resources that should be tapped.

Each segment as well as the total physical should be practiced in the laboratory with fellow students or other volunteers. Communication should be evaluated as well as the psychomotor skill level. Help in organizing the total examination, if appropriate for the program, is needed by most students. Each student needs to develop a logical sequence of examining within systems and for the total physical that is adhered to consistently.

Interpersonal skills during the physical examination

Students may master the techniques of examination but not consider the person beneath the stethoscope. Interpersonal skills do not stop with the history. The physical examination should be explained in language that can be understood by the patient (and parents of the pediatric patient) being examined. This should be demonstrated by the instructor and practiced on peers to establish a pattern of talking to the patient during the examination to explain procedures, allay anxiety, encourage questions, and continue data collection. A silent examiner with a worried look can create a poor beginning for a patient-provider relationship. In the laboratory, peers can ask what the examiner is doing and complain if the procedure hurts.

In addition to videotapes or films of the complete or partial examinations, audiotapes are available for heart and breath sounds. Several nursing and medical texts cover the content needed for obtaining a data base. (See suggested readings at the end of this chapter.)

The initial objective of teaching the physical examination is to distinguish normal from abnormal findings and to recognize and describe variations within normal. The latter is most important across age groups and should be particularly emphasized in pediatric and family nurse practitioner programs. In older adults the distinction between normal aging and pathological processes is essential.

Teaching techniques for the physical examination

Chapter 7 describes the sequence of learning psychomotor skills. The ultimate goal of learning is to be able to transfer the knowledge and skills from the clinical laboratory to wide application in caring for patients. Huckabay (1980) condensed the knowledge available on transfer of learning and listed suggestions for applying it to nursing education. Her suggestions are useful in assuring that physical examination skills are transferred to clinical situations.

1. Establish learning sets (subordinate categories of knowledge needed to perform a task).
2. Define the task or problem to the learner.
3. Increase the likelihood of attending responses to appropriate cues by focusing attention on important elements.
4. Label and identify important features of a task.
5. Maximize the similarity between the teaching situations and the ultimate testing or practice situation.
6. Provide adequate experiences with the original task.
7. Provide for a variety of examples when teaching concepts and principles.
8. Ensure that general principles are understood before expecting much transfer. (pp. 282–284).

Keeping these principles in mind and being attentive to individual differences in learning styles and tempos will promote transfer of learning from laboratory to patients and later from one patient situation to another. Efficient use of teaching resources should be a by-product of attending to learning transfer principles in that early generalization of knowledge will reduce the time and effort needed to meet objectives.

For example, transfer of learning can be facilitated in teaching the examination of the chest by several means. Cognitively, a knowledge of the anatomy of the chest and physiology of breathing is necessary. Learning sets in the psychomotor domain must also be taught before students can progress to the complete chest examination. These are inspection, palpation, percussion, and auscultation.

In breaking down the tasks still further, a variety of examples can be used to teach percussion. The wrist action is similar to the playing of staccato notes on the piano, a description that may be helpful to students who play piano. By percussing different parts of their own body (puffed cheek, thigh, jaw, abdomen) and other surfaces (over wall studs, other solid and hollow surfaces), students begin not only to acquire the ability to elicit the percussive note but also to appreciate differences in length and pitch of tones from various materials. Practice of the necessary psychomotor elements combined with presentations of didactic content teach the general principles of sound transmission from various structures rather than just the percussive note of the normal chest. Important features of the chest examination should be sequenced by lung lobes or by technique to help the student organize the examination. Later, variations for age groups and the description of abnormalities can be demonstrated on patients.

Early attention should be called to common errors such as percussing over ribs or neglecting the lateral chest walls in the examination. Omission of an element or incorrect techniques are common early in the learning of a complex task such as the chest examination and tend to be incorporated quickly. This negative learning can be minimized by very close supervision and frequent observation of practice sessions. Teaching aids such as a stethoscope with double ear pieces and an otoscope which can be used by teacher and student simultaneously help the instructor validate student findings. It is unfortunate when a student reaches the final phases of a course or program and no one has realized that errors or omissions have become part of the repertoire.

Putting it all together

As each part of the physical examination is mastered, a new teaching-learning task emerges—that of sequencing and coordinating tasks in a unified way. With adults, a head-to-toe approach has evolved but, within this format, students can develop patterns that are meaningful to them and have no omissions. Allowances are made for specific age group needs. For example, the eye, ear, nose and throat are usually the last parts examined on a toddler or early school-age child because there is discomfort and restraint is sometimes needed. Another helpful modification is having the infant or child sit on the parent's lap. (No attempt will be made here to enumerate all the tricks of the trade needed for individual clients because textbooks for specific patient groups list them.) The instructor can also pass on helpful hints from experience.

Experience has shown that a ratio of one experienced instructor to three to five students is necessary for adequate learning of physical assessment skills. A larger group can be taught by employing clinically competent nurse practitioners as assistants in the assessment laboratory.

Judicious use of all the senses, including smell, should be emphasized to obtain practice in hearing, feeling, and describing abnormalities in ambulatory settings or hospital patients. A form of hospital rounds can be employed to demonstrate abnormal physical findings that are not commonly found. Caution must be used in emphasizing the interesting and unusual so that students do not value exciting and unusual patient contacts more than the well or those with common acute and chronic problems.

Assessment and prerequisites

As more baccalaureate programs include physical assessment skills in their curricula, faculty in a nurse practitioner program may decide that knowledge of physical assessment is necessary for entrance to the program. The initial skill level of entering students must then be evaluated through some competency-based examination. Chapter 10 discusses evaluation of psychomotor skills.

Efficient use of resources

Teaching of the physical examination is expensive so that efficiency is always a consideration. What is the optimum use of audiovisual units? How much peer practice in the laboratory is needed? When well-stated behavioral criteria are met and the student voices comfort in performance of the skill, the instructor can be reasonably confident that learning has occurred. Each teaching method should reinforce previous learning but add a new stimulus. Repetition of methods can be used for individual student needs but should not be used for all students. Boredom from "overteaching" the faster students can decrease learning and motivation as much as under-teaching those with problems.

In summary, the teaching of initial data base collection can best be taught first in a laboratory setting. Use of multiple methods and adequate practice enhances learning. A suggested sequence of teaching events for each segment or system is:

1. Listing of prerequisite knowledge.
2. Presentation of objectives.
3. Viewing of video or audiotapes or films of a nurse performing the skills to be taught.
4. Talking through and demonstration of the skills by the instructor.
5. Practice of skills.
   History taking of peers or "programmed" patients.
   Physical examination of peers or models.
6. Recording of data base.
7. Evaluation.

The ability to obtain and record a history and physical examination marks the first level of expanded-role skills. This content now is included in many baccalaureate programs. Continuing education courses of two to three days' duration for registered nurses can give only an introduction to the content. Students need validation of their techniques and findings. Without an opportunity to continue practice with patients, the level of skill will deteriorate rapidly.

More depth is needed by the beginning nurse practitioner student whether in certificate, baccalaureate, or master's programs. Hence, the next step is into the real world of caring for patients.

TEACHING DIAGNOSIS AND MANAGEMENT

Diagnosis and management mark the transition from the traditional role of the nurse to becoming a primary provider of health care. This involves a combination of didactic, psychomotor, and affective education that produces a provider of primary care who can function independently and interdependently and is secure in the role. Although didactic content is taught in the classroom, application of the knowledge to patients is the final goal. The amount and type of clinical practice needed to prepare a competent provider of care is a hotly debated issue in primary care education. Many factors may play a part: beginning competencies, amount and type of supervision, and the terminal objectives of the program are the most important. It is this author's opinion that students need to see patients at least twice a week to learn and retain the necessary psychomotor skills.

The sites for teaching primary care must be chosen carefully to facilitate learning while using human and other resources efficiently. Clinical sites with attributes that facilitate student learning and that are available are rare and, when found, may already be filled with students. The ideal clinical sites for teaching expanded roles have certain physical and environmental attributes.

Physical attributes

1. Adequate number of clients.
2. A number of patients for health and illness care.
3. Adequate space and equipment for seeing patients and for conferences.
4. A heterogenous population.
5. An efficient patient flow system.
6. Ability to follow patients on return visits within the span of the course.
7. A good patient record system.

Environmental attributes

1. Qualified nurse practitioners as providers.
2. Positive staff attitudes about nurse practitioners.
3. Several professions on the health care team.
4. Positive attitudes about presence of students.

Few programs can or should use only one practice site. Depending on the purpose of the course—general primary care or specialty practice—multiple sites are usually needed to meet the objectives. Compromises and judicious combination of sites are more the rule than the exception.

Preceptor arrangements

Teaching students while faculty are engaged in their own practice has been advocated. The advantages are in efficiency, familiarity with the setting and staff, and an opportunity to serve as a practitioner role model. Disadvantages are that the instructor's relationship with patients changes with a student present and efficiency as a provider decreases. Some faculty prefer not to mix the roles of teacher and provider; others are comfortable with the combination. More often, the site will be new to the instructor as well as the students.

Arrangements for physician preception or back-up vary. A teaching team of nurse and physician faculty who have no other responsibilities while the students are present is one arrangement. The roles of each should be clear so that learning is enhanced and patients cared for adequately. A nursing faculty with considerable clinical experience can usually precept students whose patients have minor acute or chronic stable problems with minimal consultation. As problems become more complex and urgent, individual abilities dictate how much the physician is consulted. One team arrangement is for each faculty to precept half the students for a number of sessions and then exchange students. A third method is the use of physicians as back-up only for occasional consultation and for writing prescriptions in those jurisdictions where it is necessary. It is most important that physician and nurse preceptors be clinically competent as well as good teachers. The ability to teach students while the patient is present requires the highest level of clinical and teaching skill. The responsibility for review of students' records, follow-up on diagnostic procedures, and reappointment of patients must be clear so that patients' and students' needs are met.

Student anxiety

The responsibility involved in being a primary health care provider may not impact upon the student until presented with actual patients who have problems needing attention. Many students become anxious at this stage and may "regress" even though their performance in the laboratory was successful. To overcome this professional identity crisis, the instructor can structure clinical experience for optimum learning by:

- adequate orientation
- making expectations clear
- making realistic and appropriate assignments
- assigning patients with problems covered in classroom teaching
- being available for guidance
- encouraging independence
- giving adequate feedback often

The crisis that comes with the first real patient's management is detailed in Chapter 2. The concern about becoming a "mini-doc" is a healthy sign that, once the medical skills are learned, they can be integrated into an expanded nursing role.

Orientation

Student orientation includes mundane but necessary information such as provisions for parking, lockers, cafeteria, proper dress, introduction to staff, and tour of the facility. A talk-through of a clinical period also decreases anxiety. Just as adult learners have different cognitive styles, they also adapt to new environments at different rates and with diverse coping mechanisms.

Expectations can be communicated through formal written objectives but a discussion of roles, lines of authority, and agency practices and policies are helpful. Students should know if there will be a time limit for seeing patients and if they will be observed and by whom. Worry about evaluation of clinical performance should be alleviated by handing out the evaluation tool to be used early in the course. Chapter 10 discusses methods for student evaluation.

Patient assignments

Patients should be assigned that are appropriate to the student's ability and the course objectives. It is often impossible, particularly early in the course, to make a perfect selection. If the didactic material has not yet been covered, students can be led through some on-the-spot problem solving based on their previous nursing experience. Having a good reference library close by facilitates learning. For an illness visit, one patient in a two to three hour period may be all that a new student can manage well. As the course or program progresses, efficiency must increase to meet real-world expectations. Emphasis in teaching shifts from completeness to setting priorities and focusing on the goal(s) for the particular visit. Pediatric students seeing well children or those students in a specialty facility (i.e., women's health, hypertension) may be able to see more patients in a given time than those sites where patients have a number of chronic or acute problems.

When clients do not appear for appointments, the flexibility of the instructor is tested. One commonly used technique is the assignment of two students to one client. This can be potentially overwhelming for the patient and/or wasteful of students' time without careful planning. Methods of making dual assignments are described in Chapter 9.

"Down time" can also be used to teach laboratory techniques. A willing laboratory technician or the instructor can demonstrate urinalysis, blood smears, gram stains, and vaginal smears. Students can then practice without the pressure of a patient waiting.

Another technique when there is a shortage of patients is the clinical conference, formally or informally conducted. The experience of one student can benefit others when a case from the previous day is analyzed. If the instructor notes a learning deficit in several students, a group discussion with prior preparation is helpful. Even with adequate classroom preparation, transfer of learning to clinical situations may not occur without presenting the content in several ways or making special assignments. Because of differences in previous clinical nursing experience this occurs more frequently at the continuing education and graduate level.

Availability of clients to illustrate all major content areas for each student is rare. More often other means must be used to provide comparable experience. Chapter 9 discusses the use of simulation, professional patients, and computer-assisted instruction which can be used to present case studies for practice in diagnosis and management.

Follow-up

Follow-up visits are necessary to provide an opportunity to evaluate the prescribed management regime. This is facilitated by having a defined goal from the previous visit. Not only should the nurse practitioner student ask whether the medication or treatment worked but also what the patient knows about the problem. Students can be taught to evaluate both the process and outcome of care. Outcome is the "bottom line" but looking at process may help explain the outcome. Having to replan with new goals may humble a student and emphasize the complex art of providing care. Follow-up visits also provide opportunities for sequential teaching and establishing a long-term patient-provider relationship.

Referral

An aspect of teaching management of patient care is the decision to consult with or to refer to colleagues. New practitioners will consult and refer more often than more experienced ones. Either over-referral or underreferral is not cost-effective or in the patient's best interest. An example of overreferral would be for a nurse practitioner to refer to a health educator or nutritionist for routine counseling. Referral should ordinarily be to another provider who has more expertise for further diagnosis or management of a particular problem, but referrals can also be made to move a patient to a less expensive system for his particular needs. Helping the student assess strengths and deficits can have far-reaching results so that proper consultation and referral are done as a graduate.

Teaching the diagnostic process

Diagnosis is essentially a problem-solving process, the highest cognitive level according to Gagne (1965). The steps in the problem solving process are:

1. Identification of the problem.
2. Selecting alternative solutions.
3. Evaluating outcomes of the selected alternatives.

4. Choosing one or more solutions.
5. Evaluating the outcome.

The parallel steps in the nursing process of assessment, planning, implementation, and evaluation can be pointed out. In essence, the nursing process and medical diagnosis are specific applications of the problem-solving process. Problems are identified from the data base, alternative and appropriate solutions are selected and evaluated, and one or more treatment measures initiated. On later visits the outcome is evaluated and treatment modified as necessary.

Students have various difficulties at each step. They may not recognize the existence of abnormal findings with the physical or in the history. In this event, the instructor can suggest a review of the normative findings for the particular client.

In evaluating the data base for problem identification, some students are overwhelmed and unable to synthesize the information. Focus can be provided by the instructor through asking specific questions. Commitment to one's diagnosis should be encouraged once the data has been synthesized. If an incorrect diagnosis is made, pointing out missing data or errors in logic must be done in a constructive manner.

Where algorithms or protocols are used, the student does not have the opportunity to develop a logic tree for diagnosis. Experience in other sites where they are not used is necessary to help students develop their own problem-solving ability.

The fine art of diagnosis

As mentioned before, diagnosis is little more than the identification of problems, a task well known in nursing. The new aspect is the expansion from nursing problems or diagnosis to total health and illness problems. The mass of information obtained in the data base must be sorted out, summarized, and evaluated. The result is a list of the clients' health care problems. Initially, students can do little more than list each deviation from normal in the data base. Then with help they can inductively combine data to identify more complex problems. For instance, a beginning student might list the abnormal findings for a 45-year-old woman as: (1) moist skin; (2) nervousness; (3) insomnia; and (4) resting heart rate of 100/minute. This cluster of symptoms and signs would lead an experienced provider to suspect a thyroid dysfunction and order the proper diagnostic tests. However, a beginning student must be led through the logic of listing all possible causes for such abnormalities and weighing the probability of each before synthesizing a diagnosis.

The next step is to set priorities. Not all problems must be diagnosed and treated at the first visit. If this is a new patient with several problems, the most pressing—as determined by both the student and the patient—is pursued. After this is accomplished, a contract with the patient can be made for further attention to less pressing problems.

There is a tendency for new students in expanded roles to neglect the identification and "treatment" of psychosocial problems, a strength of most nurses. The nursing instructor can support the need to concentrate on the new skills of identifying medical problems, but should also remind the student to assess clients holistically.

Teaching patient management

The step of deciding treatment modalities is another that is new for many nurses. Although they may have played the doctor-nurse game by leading physicians to a diagnosis and treatment decision, the final responsibility was not theirs. The instructor can help students identify possible treatment modalities, evaluate their use, and make a choice. Students who find it difficult to tolerate ambiguity may become distressed when they discover that, for most health and illness care, there is often no clear-cut management decision even for patients with the same problem. These students sometimes feel the instructor is clinically indecisive rather than recognize that several alternatives may be equally viable. Also needing help is the student who is disorganized and cannot sort out the important findings or make the most obvious diagnosis.

The match between instructor and student is important when a learning problem arises. One advantage of the nurse-physician preceptor team is the flexibility it offers to the student. Often someone who does not know a student's past history can facilitate learning more than one who has had previous difficulties with the student and may prejudge behavior in a new situation.

THE ART OF PRECEPTING

Guidance of nursing students at any level is more an art than a science. Individual needs for support and information must be met but it is helpful to step back occasionally and consider whether some students should be encouraged to solve problems more independently. Questioning to determine knowledge level of the pathophysiology, diagnosis, and management of a problem helps the students recall and validate knowledge or identity areas needing further study. Some faculty prefer to use a Socratic method of questioning, commonly used in medical and law education (see Chapter 7). Other instructors are comfortable with a more gentle approach combining questioning and affirmation. Clinical skills of faculty are a factor in guidance. Chapter 3 elaborates the importance of faculty development of clinical expertise. However, nursing or medical faculty should not conceal their own need for seeking consultation or using references. In fact, this is an aspect of role modeling that demonstrates to students the use of resources and the ability to refer or consult when necessary. Students will pick up subtle behaviors of the nurse preceptor. If the role message is not clear, students may indeed begin to model the physician's behavior. Both need to be comfortable with their roles and use confrontation without hostility when disagreements in patient management occur.

Feedback and evaluation

Because faculty are in clinical sites for most expanded-role courses, there is a tendency to assume that students are made aware of their performance level and abilities. However, it is important to provide a time for periodic formal oral or written evaluation of clinical performance. A daily, brief evaluation is preferable but is often lost in the press of time to dispense patients or get to class. A time should be set up for individual conferences to evaluate strengths and weaknesses mutually.

Other assignments

Other teaching techniques can enhance what is learned from patient care. Written assignments help to analyze clinical situations more leisurely than is possible in the clinical site. Complete data bases and SOAP (episodic) notes can be copied and rewritten as an exercise in self-assessment. Case histories can be used to provide additional experience in essential content or the unusual clinical situations. Computer-assisted learning, programmed instruction, construction of algorithms or protocols, and production of patient education materials are all methods of helping the student synthesize and apply knowledge to clinical situations. Some of these are covered in greater detail in Chapter 9 on creative teaching methods.

PRESENTATION AND RECORDING OF DATA

The task of presenting findings to a colleague or preceptor is important to the concept of the team approach to care. Data must be organized, synthesized, and presented so that the essential facts are emphasized and communicated to others through the patient's record. Students should be given a format to follow. The Weed or SOAP system is commonly used for both presentation and recording. All aspects of the history (chief complaint, history of present illness, past medical history, family history, review of systems) are included in the subjective data. Physical findings and laboratory x-ray results are presented in the objective data. The most likely assessment (diagnosis or problem) is given first but with attention to other likely possibilities. The plan includes treatment modalities, further diagnostic procedures, and patient education (Weed, 1971). Some providers also include a goal or goals for the next visit.

The oral presentation is a stressful event for most students. Practice with peers may ease the anxiety but each preceptor may have peculiarities that require flexibility. Students must have encouragement to support and defend their decision but, at the same time, to acknowledge missing data and deficits in knowledge.

For legal purposes and communicating to others, recording of data is needed. Because of this and, for some, because of difficulties in writing, it produces undue anxiety in some students. Despite extensive experience in writing nurses' notes, few students have read in detail or critiqued a written data base. If they have, most are poor examples. Again, the Weed method is a common format used. Agency modifications are common and should be made known to the students. Whatever format is selected, students need written guidelines or a sample data base. In Appendix I of this book are examples of both complete and episodic notes for several hypothetical patients. Adequate practice, early and often, with written and oral feedback will help to establish patterns of accurate and complete recording. Criterion-referenced grading seems most appropriate for the data base. Attention to use of correct and appropriate terminology, spelling, and the recording of pertinent negatives will indicate the degree of precision needed to communicate a data base to others as well as for legal purposes.

MOVING TOWARD INDEPENDENCE

Most expanded-role programs include a final practicum or apprenticeship period. This experience is characterized by:

1. Working directly with health team members.
2. Polishing assessment, diagnosis, and management skills.
3. Working with a defined population in one setting.
4. Increased clinical time.
5. Follow-up of patients.
6. Increasing efficiency.
7. Working without direct, continuous supervision.

The benefits of having a transition to the work world are obvious. Reality shock for nurse practitioners in their first jobs is as critical as for new RNs (Kramer, 1974). Some of the shock comes when they are expected to see a certain number of patients per day or there is a demand for skills not taught in the basic practitioner program. A number of these expectations and problems of acceptance of the expanded role in the clinical site can be faced with the help of instructors who should visit the site periodically. Conferences or seminars with fellow students from other clinical placements provide opportunities to discuss common practice issues.

Instructors should negotiate the placement as with earlier clinical placements, giving particular attention to meeting individual student needs. Students may prefer a specialty clinic, a particular population, type of institution (school, industry, clinic), or level of care (acute, chronic, health maintenance). Some return to their previous practice site before entering the program. Only one student should be present in a site at a time to receive full benefit of the placement. If two students are placed together there is often a tendency to rely on each other rather than integrating themselves into the staff.

Together the student and instructor can evaluate readiness for the preferred site. In addition to the general clinical objectives, students can plan to remedy deficits and develop new skills. Instructor visits are used for observation and conferencing with the student and selected staff members. One person—a nurse practitioner or physician—should be identified to provide direct supervision and input to evaluation. Placement in a solo practice simplifies communication, but also may carry the risk of providing a narrower experience than a group practice.

Classmates become a peer support group to compare and discuss experiences. If all didactic and clinical content has been presented prior to the final practicum, some of the more complex professional and clinical issues such as third party reimbursement, clinical privileges for nurse practitioners, and political forces on practice can be explored in the apprenticeship period.

Students should spend one or more full days or evenings in the clinical site to become integrated into the staff, socialized further into the role, and to become familiar with policies and procedures.

SUMMARY

This chapter has presented techniques and a sequence for clinical teaching in the expanded role. Eliciting and recording the complete data base in a laboratory setting using teacher demonstration, audiovisual aids, and practice on peers or models is the initial step. These skills can then be transferred to working with patients in health screening or nonacute settings. As diagnosis and management knowledge and skills are added through didactic and clinical teaching, the students take on the role of a primary care provider. Roles of nurse and physician faculty preceptors and negotiation of clinical sites were discussed.

REFERENCES

Bloom, B. S. (Ed.)., *Taxonomy of educational objectives. Handbook I: Cognitive domain*. New York: Longmans, Inc., 1977.

Bridgman, C. F. & Suter, E. Searching AVLINE for curriculum related audiovisual instructional material. *Journal of Medical Education*, 1979, *54*, 236–337.

Gagne, R. M. *The conditions of learning*. New York: Holt, Rinehart & Winston, 1965.

Huckabay, L. M. D. *Conditions of learning and instruction in nursing*. Saint Louis: C. V. Mosby Company, 1980.

Jones, C. Negotiating student placements in ambulatory settings. *Journal of Nursing Education*, 1983, *25*, (6), 255–258.

Knafl, K. A. How real is the practicum for nurse practitioner students? *Nursing Outlook*, 1979, *27*, (2), 131–135.

Kramer, M. *Reality shock: Why nurses leave nursing*. Saint Louis: C. V. Mosby Company, 1974.

Sparks, S. M., Vitalo, P. B., Cohen, B. F., & Kahn, G. S. Teaching of interpersonal skills to nurse practitioner students. *Journal of Continuing Education in Nursing*, 1980, *11*, 5–16.

Weed, L. L. *Medical records, medical education, and patient care: The problem-oriented records as a basic tool*. Cleveland: Case Western Reserve University Press, 1971.

SUGGESTED READINGS

Bates, B. *A guide to physical examination*, 3rd ed. Philadelphia: J. B. Lippincott Company, 1983.

Bates, B. & Lynaugh, J. Teaching physical assessment. *Nursing Outlook*, 1975, *23*, 297–302.

Benjamin, A. *The helping interview*, 3rd ed. Boston: Houghton Mifflin, 1981.

Bevil, C. W. .& Gross, L. C. Assessing the adequacy of clinical learning centers. *Nursing Outlook*, 1981, *29*, 658–661.

Brammer, L. M. *The helping relationship: Process and skills*, 2nd ed. Englewood Cliffs, New Jersey: Prentice-Hall, 1979.

Burns, K. R. & Johnson, P. J. *Health assessment in clinical practice*. Englewood Cliffs, New Jersey: Prentice-Hall, 1980.

DeGowin, E. L. & DeGowin, R. L. *Bedside Diagnostic Examination*, 4th ed. Macmillan, New York, 1981.

Garrett, A. M. *Interviewing: Its principles and methods*, 3rd ed. New York: Family Service Association of America, 1982.

Gillies, D. A. & Alyn, I. B. *Patient assessment and management by the nurse practitioner*. Philadelphia: W. B. Saunders Company, 1976.

Mahoney, E. A. & Verdisco, L. A. *How to collect and record a health history*. Philadelphia: J. B. Lippincott, 1982.

Malassanos, E. L., Barkauskas, V., Moss, M., & Stoltenberg-Allen, K. *Health assessment*, 2nd ed. Saint Louis: C. V. Mosby Company, 1981.

O'Shea, H. S. & Parsons, M. K. Clinical instruction: Effective/and ineffective teacher behaviors. *Nursing Outlook*, 1979, *27*, 411–415.

Prior, J. A., Silberstein, J. S., & Stang, J. M. *Physical diagnosis: The history and examination of the patient*, 6th ed. Saint Louis: C. V. Mosby Company, 1981.

Quarto, J. M. & Natapoff, J. N. Health maintenance and physical assessment skills in baccaluareate programs in New York State: A pilot study. *Journal of the New York State Nurses' Association, 10* (3), 9–13.

Rasendow, A. M. Helping practitioner students put concepts into action. *Nursing Outlook*, 1977, *25*, (7), 446–449.

Siegel, H. J. & Elsberry, N. Master's preparation for joint practice. *Nursing Outlook*, 1979, *27*, (1), 57–60.

9

Other Teaching Methodologies

Marilyn Winterton Edmunds

The use of the classroom lecture and the clinical assignment experience remain standard and irreplaceable parts of teaching methodology. However, use of innovative techniques to enhance the lecture, including development of unusual methodologies of presentation and creative student assignments, do much to increase the learning that takes place. Experiences which "come alive" will often be remembered indefinitely by students if they are stimulating enough. Specific points, a philosophical viewpoint, and major concepts may all be taught in a way which maximizes learning and increases retention.

The gamut of teaching strategies runs from the use of simple audiovisual slides or overhead transparencies to the construction of elaborate faculty dramas, or use of simulated patient encounters. A parallel spectrum also exists for methodologies which are inexpensive, which require substantial financial outlay, those which are easy to prepare, and those which need complex and time-consuming development. A listing of some strategies which might be adopted for classroom use, for clinical use, and as assignments to guide the student learning can be seen in Table 9-1.

This chapter is designed to provide a brief examination of selected strategies which have special merit for nurse practitioner programs. Specific examples are provided where possible to demonstrate practical and realistic application of suggestions.

Table 9-1. Creative Teaching Methodologies

CLASSROOM TEACHING METHODOLOGIES

Audio-Visual Slides
Transparencies
Movies
    Demonstration of Techniques
    Teaching of Content
Faculty Role-Playing
Student Role-Playing
Problem Negotiation
Games
        Card Games
        Board Games
        Active Games
Faculty Drama

STUDENT ASSIGNMENTS

Computer-Assisted Instruction
Role Assumption
Algorithms
Protocols
Marketing Portfolio Development
Audits
Lesson Plans
Flip Chart Development
Writing Booklets
Programmed Instruction
Script Writing
Video Productions

CLINICAL TEACHING ASSIGNMENTS

Patient Simulations
Paid Patients
Dual Student Patient Assignments
Student Audit
In-Patient Hospital Rounds
Audio-Taping
Video-Taping of Student-Client Interactions

WHY OTHER METHODOLOGIES ARE USEFUL

Goals of education

In the past, the cost of educating health care personnel has always been substantial. This has continued to be the rule for nurse practitioner programs as well. Because of the densely packed content in the brief programs, and the need for careful clinical supervision (requiring low faculty-student ratios in order to ascertain the safety of nurse practitioner performance), use of creative teaching methods is one way to reduce the enormous expense of educating nurse practitioners. Methods which decrease direct faculty time (i.e., videotaping client-student interactions for later viewing), maximize student time, or utilize one patient encounter for many students' learning experiences are all ways of decreasing direct or indirect costs for the program.

Need to maximize resources

In addition to decreasing costs, a parallel reason for using different strategies is the obvious need to maximize resources. Academic program faculty, patients, and students are struggling financially in the contemporary health care scene. Abuse or wasting of the time of any of these three groups of people jeopardizes the longevity of any program.

Patients are a particularly valuable resource. They may not always be available when needed for students, or not in sufficient numbers for each student to be with one patient. It is sometimes difficult to find patients with particular diagnoses with which students should have some experience. And it is always a problem to correlate patient experiences with content which is being presented in the classroom. Dual student assignments to a patient, use of in-hospital patient rounds, hiring of "simulated" patients, or use of computerized cases may strengthen a program in particular patient need areas.

Preceptors are another valuable resource. They are usually one of the more expensive components of a curriculum. The need for experienced preceptors who can work with a variety of personalities, with students at varying levels of development and experience, and who can teach as well as evaluate are always sought. Preceptors need to be present constantly to validate student findings and learning. There should be sufficient numbers of both nursing and physician preceptors so that there can be a "fit" component of the role, and to establish proper role models. Because preceptors are so expensive to hire, maximum utilization of their time must be ensured.

Time is another valuable resource which can be saved by careful teaching strategies. Time in the clinical areas can be planned to anticipate slow time while students wait for patients or preceptors. Planned activities such as learning to do laboratory work or use of in-patient rounds can be instituted when there is a lack of patients. One student assignment might be used as a base for multiple requirements to save students from repeating work.

Methodologies should also be planned to take advantage of existing equipment owned by a nurse practitioner program, or which can be purchased with long-term use in mind. Often development of videotapes or audio-recordings preserves excellent lectures if a program cannot hire these same lectures to be given more than once. Investment in valuable software which can be used repeatedly to demonstrate key components of the program is also wise. Sometimes exceptional students need extra challenges, or another student may need remedial help in an area. Computerized patient cases may provide assistance for both these types of students, or supplement areas in which all students need more exposure.

Stimulation for student and teacher

A third major benefit in using a variety of teaching strategies comes in direct stimulation to both the teacher and the student. Innovative strategies allow the instructor to do something different with content which is repeated each year. Many strategies give encouragement to both the creative student and instructor and both benefit from this freedom. Often the nurse practitioner student is a very talented, creative person, willing to do things differently and take risks. (That is probably one reason they have chosen to be in the nurse practitioner role!) These are the people who respond well to opportunities to use their own ideas and initiative in expressing themselves. Use of a variety of types of student assignments provides additional ways of assessing student performance, especially for students who may not do as well on traditional forms of testing.

Add "wow" to the program

A final reason for using a cornucopia of nontraditional teaching methodologies is as a way to add sparkle to the program content. Specific activities that create memories aid retention of material and can change a good program into an outstanding program. Activities that stimulate faculty often cause a feeling of enthusiasm which is contagious to the students. Both faculty and students should feel part of a dynamic curriculum, in which their own individual personalities can play a part. The creative student can obtain visibility which brings positive rewards. Many faculty ideas develop naturally into articles or books, which can then be published. This is a healthy spirit in academia which should be encouraged, rather than the sickly "publish or perish" mentality which is so prevalent.

WHEN ADDITIONAL TEACHING STRATEGIES ARE USEFUL

In the early stages of the program, specific techniques might be used as a way of orienting the student to what will be expected in the program. Some strategies can be used as a way of demonstrating something in particular the student is to do, and specifically how it is to be done. For example, faculty might show a video-tape of how history taking might be conducted in several different types of patient encounters: What is asked the first time the nurse practitioner sees a patient and is collecting a complete data base; taking a screening history; doing a follow-up on an episodic problem.

As the student progresses in the program, replay of sequentially-taped audio and video recordings are an excellent way for faculty and students to monitor progress. Documentation of this student progress is also helpful to the instructor for grading purposes, for collecting program evaluation material, or for specific research purposes.

STRATEGIES FOR STIMULATING
THE STUDENT DIRECTLY

In actively challenging students to learn through creative teaching, the basic purpose is to require them to organize required content in a new way. This is particularly true when students must review content in the classroom, which they may be familiar with already from their previous nursing role. Building new methods upon an existing foundation is a way of expanding the knowledge students already have to new situations. Sometimes a creative teaching strategy asks students to take material which they learn in textbooks or lecture and use it immediately. This allows students to "handle" content intimately and fully process it cognitively. Putting ideas into their own words or a new format allows students to test out material they have learned and reflect it back in another manner. Thus the adequacy of learning can be evaluated.

The outcome to be achieved when "stimulating" techniques are utilized is increased student involvement in the learning process itself. Whenever the student is involved directly, the activity becomes not just another assignment, but something that touches them as individuals. Assignments then can be personalized by student creativity and perspective. Students can also shape assignments to focus on the things they do the best, giving them numerous opportunities to perform and to succeed in the program. For example, perhaps a student is also a talented artist. Giving this student freedom in an assignment might allow her to use her artistic skills in displaying the material she needs to know.

Examples of specific student assignments especially helpful in stimulating nurse practitioner students will be briefly mentioned. (See Table 9-2 for a listing of these creative student assignments.)

Algorithms

The student is asked to construct a detailed "decision-tree" pertaining to a given symptom or problem. The student must determine at least five or six pertinent questions to ask the patient about the problem. The "yes" or "no" responses to the questions determine what question should be asked next, what laboratory work should be done, or what

Table 9-2.   Student Assignments Designed to "Stimulate"

Construction of Algorithms

Writing of Protocols

Development of Programmed Instruction Panels

Development of Criteria and Audits

Script Writing and Production

Lesson Plan Development

Creation of Patient-Teaching Flip-Charts

Development of Patient-Education Booklets

Video-Tape of Student Performances

---

teaching should be done. The end result is the answer to "what needs to be done today?"

Writing an algorithm is a disciplined exercise in logic. They are highly organized and directive, yet involve the patient intimately in their implementation. Students are required to master a good deal of knowledge. Questions must be written which will yield the precise information the student needs in order to go on to the next level of decision making. Consideration of past history, discovery of major signs and symptoms, and establishment of a differential diagnosis are all items which must be pursued. Specific teaching or treatments are then planned dependent upon answers that are given to each question.

Protocols

In contrast to algorithms, protocols are formats which identify either the ideal or the required procedure in dealing with the total scope of a particular problem. For a selected diagnosis, the student is required to clearly determine what information must be asked in the history, what findings to look for during the physical exam, what diagnostic work should be done, as well as correct management for a diagnosed problem.

Protocols are designed to provide a data base which will be consistent, to help achieve thoroughness, and to facilitate audit of care. In addition, a protocol should be convenient to use, and lead to continued learning whenever possible (Hudak, Redstone, Hokanson, & Suzuki, 1976).

Protocols are gaining increasing popularity, especially in sites where nurse practitioners may not always have physician coverage. Because they have been called "recipes" by some critics, students must be aware of the rigidity with which some protocols are used so that other coexisting patient problems or behavior may make modifications imperative.

Because of the increase in use of protocols, there are now numerous published examples which students might evaluate and critique which will help them both in their own attempts to write proposals, and in their wise approach to their future use in practice.

Programmed instruction

The ability to write a programmed instruction panel is a sophisticated skill which should be saved for the more advanced graduate student interested in teaching. This activity is excellent for a student who has done outstanding work on a case presentation or classroom assignment which may merit publication. It is mandatory, if a student plans to spend the time involved in doing a project of this nature, that the subject matter be carefully narrowed down. If possible, they should also receive special assistance from someone with a background in writing programmed instruction.

Developing criteria for audits

As nurse practitioner students begin to give care to patients they rapidly discover the difficulty in recording all the important dimensions of the patient encounter. As writeups of care are evaluated by different preceptors, it is obvious that they are examined from a variety of viewpoints—sometimes seemingly contradictory. An exercise to formalize criteria to audit a record may help the student understand the wide variety of ways a record can be written and still be acceptable. A record might meet the criteria for "comprehensiveness" but fail against a criteria for "accuracy." Unless criteria are specified, it is difficult to learn principles which can be generalized to all record keeping.

Script writing and production

Another assignment which stimulates creative thinking and artistry involves taking a common teaching assignment which nurse practitioners might engage in with a client and developing it into a formal script. For example, explaining to a patient who has a urinary tract infection "what it is," "what should be done to treat it," and "how to decrease chances of reinfection" might be developed into a five-minute presentation. Perhaps a short sequence explaining to a cardiac patient how nitro paste is properly applied might be written. These common teaching sessions can also be produced using cartoons, role-playing, or words with graphic displays, and videotapes. The content could then be shown to patients when specifically needed, or used in the curriculum to support or illustrate lectures. The main learning experience comes from actually determining what has to be said for a given problem, how to say it, and how it can be displayed in a method that promotes patient learning.

Lesson plans/flip-charts/booklets

Using the same content as presented in a video-taped script, material might be organized as a lesson plan (defining objectives for content to be taught, activities to support content, and how evaluation of learning takes place). Content might also be developed into a flip-chart to use in teaching patients in an office, or as booklets which might be duplicated so patients can take them home.

A group of these items can be developed by each class within a program, with each succeeding class getting ideas from previously completed projects. It only takes a few years to have a rich library of student-created supplemental teaching tools for students to share with each other and with patients.

STRATEGIES FOR INCREASING
STUDENT INVOLVEMENT IN LEARNING

It is well-documented that most students relate easier to assignments about which they have some personal experience or knowledge. Several leading authorities (Russell, 1974; Dale, 1969) suggest that next to actual experiences, physical involvement with artificial or simulated experiences is the most valuable form of learning.

A major group of activities designed to personally stimulate students are the "life-practice" strategies. The purpose of these activities is to present information and to involve the student personally by practicing real behaviors in a simulated situation. Life-practice strategies then require the student to actively demonstrate components of either the nurse practitioner role, or the patient role.

In order to be better able to counsel patients with particular experiences, the student may "assume" a particular problem, become emotionally involved with it, and develop a perspective from the patient's point of view.

Because students don't have opportunities to work with all the patient problems which would be desirable in a program, role assumption is also a way of compensating for less than desirable resources. Not everyone can care for a patient who has been raped, or a mother who has a still-born baby. Simulation of these problems may help fill in gaps in student experiences, or round out a curriculum which has a skewed patient population because of particular clinical sites used. (For example, a program that uses primarily geriatric sites may have students who lack adequate family planning experiences.)

Sometimes the role is assumed by a faculty member rather than a student as a way of maximizing a teaching-learning situation. This may be a mechanism for allowing several students to become involved in one problem. Sometimes by making an experience so startling, repetition (which is often needed to cause retention of information) will not be necessary. Thus complex faculty drama may be a valuable teaching tool also.

Examples of specific life-practice strategies will be mentioned, and a listing of these techniques can be found in Table 9-3.

Table 9-3. Sample of "Life-Practice" Strategies

Role Assumption

        Living With A Chronic Disease
        Undergoing Surgery
        Special Diets
        Rape
        Death In The Family
        Divorce
        Terminal Illness In The Family
        Infertility-Adoption
        Assignment "On-Wheels"

Disaster Evacuation Drama

Problem Negotiation

Marketing Portfolio Development and Job Interview Practice

Professional Patients

        Pre-and Post-Course Evaluations
        Provide "Intimate" Exam Experience

Computer-Assisted Learning

Video-Taping Student Interactions With Clients

Role-Playing

        By Faculty
        By Students

"Focusing" Students in Clinical Experiences

        Dual Student Assignments
        Use of Criterion-Referenced Evaluation

Audit Activities

        Self-Audit
        Peer Audit

Role assumption

In this activity the student is required to "assume" the problem or situation of someone else. The student is assigned a particular role for a defined period of time. This may be for a brief period of time, or it may last for an entire semester, as students learn about a sustained problem and its evolution.

Some of the following "roles" can be used for student assignments, with very obvious and direct learning outcomes.

Life problems experienced with chronic disease. For example, give students a diagnosis of "high blood pressure," along with a prescription for medications. Students must go to several pharmacies, comparatively price medications, and then actually take candy "pills" as their prescription dictates. The most important component of the activity is the follow-up discussion about why students don't comply with this assignment: "Too busy," "not real," "too expensive," "inconvenient," "forgot." These same problems exist in real life and are the reasons patients don't comply. Patients often don't feel "ill."

Surgery (for example, hernia repair, abortion, having a baby). Prepare students by giving them a diagnosis. Have them go to a hospital, prepare for surgery by making arrangements with the operating room staff to talk with students in the evening, finding out what will happen preoperatively, what they are told will happen, where they will go during surgery and after surgery, what will happen to them specifically, how visitors/family can reach them, amount of pain, nausea, and so on. What is the reputation of the surgeons involved? What complications might be expected? What do hospital staff do which may help or hinder this surgery?

Special diets. Assign students to go on a special diet: American Diabetic Association (ADA) diet, low sodium, or a combination. Maintain this diet for a specified time. Keep a record of problems with the diet. Talk about why they do not comply, and how this is important in counseling patients. What new knowledge is gained from personal experience?

Rape. Students are to assume they have been raped. Faculty members will make arrangements so they can go to an emergency room and talk to doctors, nurses, rape counselor, police, as well as talk with their husbands, boyfriends, or minister about their feelings about rape. Discover what support groups are available. What facilities, help centers, what problems can be anticipated, and how to deal with them. Share with classmates, in the form of a booklet, material which has been found. Include things that might be helpful or not helpful to someone who has recently been raped.

Death in the family. Wife suddenly loses husband. Student must discover what must be done: funeral arrangements and expenses; will vs. no will; probate; taxes. What does it cost? What support groups are there? What will be the problems for someone newly widowed? What is helpful? Not helpful?

Divorce. Assume husband suddenly (with no advance warning) says he wants a divorce. What are your legal rights? How does a divorce proceed? How long does it take in your state? What are the grounds? What is the expense involved? What support groups are there? What problems might be anticipated?

Terminal illness in the family. Parents have been told that their child has leukemia, with a long-term but eventually fatal course. What stresses are to be anticipated? What options are available? What issues must be dealt with? Are there support groups to help with these stressors?

Infertility/Adoption. Assume that you and your spouse have been trying to have children for several years. Ascertain what constitutes an infertility workup for both men and women. When is a workup indicated? What pressures will be felt by both men and women? Are there support systems for this problem? Assume you have no children. Investigate laws pertaining to and the methods available for adoption. Make this situation specific to your state and county. What are the expenses in adoption? The problems to be faced when you do or do not obtain a child to adopt?

Assignment "on-wheels". An instructor, herself confined to a wheelchair, developed the idea of having students spend at least a day on campus in a wheelchair. They were required to go about their normal activities, but needed to go into at least two different buildings on campus, and to a restroom in one building. Students wrote a paper about their experiences, identifying physical barriers, as well as psychological difficulties encountered in overcoming the problem of having restricted mobility.

Disaster evacuation

Another type of dramatic life-problem simulation can be developed around disaster techniques. Military personnel are often willing to donate time and facilities to help students develop practical skills in disaster nursing. Students can prepare components of the lecture content, and are told they will be called upon to teach others the material without advance warning or preparation. Class members can then be awakened at 4:30 a.m. and told to "evacuate" to a campus building with a blanket. Students can remain on campus or could be further "evacuated" to an army base for a three-day disaster training. Students are required to prepare and eat dehydrated survival food. Emergency courses are presented by the students when indicated for "patients" they find who have broken bones, burns, drowning, have multiple injuries and need to be moved, or go into labor and need emergency deliveries. Emotional problems common in mass disaster situations can also be simulated, along with ways of dealing with them. Invitation of the public media to cover this three-day course adds some excitement to a high-tension learning period. Students preparing to become emergency nurse practitioners would profit most from this or a less elaborate disaster simulation.

Problem negotiation

This is a technique borrowed from conflict management theory, in which conflict is reduced and agreement reached through a process of negotiation. For example, a nurse practitioner and a "patient" need to agree on which patient problems should be pursued as they work together in an out-patient setting. The nurse practitioner feels that some behaviors (i.e., smoking, having no job) are problems. The patient does not want to worry about these things, but wants some medication for insomnia. Each party to this disagreement about the problems to be pursued writes on a separate card each problem which they see as important, and then stacks the cards in the order of priority for resolution. Then the two people sit down together to examine how each has listed and prioritized problems. The two parties must talk about the problems and the priorities until they can both agree on one stack of problems and the priorities in which they should be approached. This technique clearly emphasizes the need for patient involvement in determining what assistance the patient requires from the nurse practitioner (Edmunds, 1979).

Marketing portfolio and job interview practice

Students assemble a "marketing portfolio" made up of all the items they would need in order to apply for a job: a resume or curriculum vitae, a position description for a job they desire, copy of current licensure and malpractice insurance, abstract of thesis, copy of articles they may have written, sample history and physical examination, sample lesson plans, copies of booklets they may have developed for teaching patients, and so on. They also write a letter of inquiry about a particular position. This portfolio can be critiqued by students and faculty. Then students take turns interviewing each other for a job, and evaluating the "prospective applicant" upon defined parameters of their interview performance. Specific comments are given to help them prepare for their first real job interview (Edmunds, 1980).

Use of professional patients

Professional patients, or simulated patient encounters, have been an accepted strategy in medical schools for years. "The limited evidence available suggests that well designed instruction and evaluative simulations may be more effective than clinical instruction based on real patients at the initial skill development stage" (Maatsch, 1979).

Because nurses initially come to nurse practitioner programs with a variety of past experiences and skills, it is often unclear where to begin teaching a class of students. It is not even possible to generalize from one class of students to another. Even students themselves don't always have the ability to know whether their skills are adequate or not. In a research study in progress, no correlation could be found between the students' personal evaluation of their ability to perform a history and physical, and their objectively graded performance doing a history and physical examination. (Some students overrate their ability; some underrate themselves.) Taking time to bring in a professional patient with known history and physical findings for the student to interview and examine is a useful way of determining actual student competence. Repeating the process at the end of a semester may help determine what learning has actually taken place and define areas of strength and weakness in both students and the curriculum or teaching methodologies.

Use of pre- and post-performance evaluation techniques has several major requirements. The first and most important is the necessity of having objective criteria developed in order to document how a student is performing. It cannot be subjective, or findings are really not conclusive. The second requirement is to teach a group of people to serve as "simulated patients." Sometimes actors can be hired. Often other students within the program will volunteer to be patients. The "patients" must be primed: given complaints, symptoms, and a history of present illness. They must be taught how to be patients. They often feel very guilty, and feel like they are lying to the student interviewing them. They want so much to help students, and it bothers them when students get side-tracked in the history and never focus upon the correct information. The best "patients" are usually those who are hired, and have no vested interest in the student's performance, but this is often a more expensive proposition.

A second opportunity for use of paid or simulated patients might occur when students need practice performing more intimate examinations before they try them with real patients. Usually the greatest difficulty in finding practice experience comes in learning to do pelvic, rectal, and prostate examinations. Students have more reluctance about doing these examinations on patients than any other component of the physical examination. They feel they are exploiting patients when they practice an intimate examination, but not when they practice a chest examination. Some programs have hired individuals to allow students to obtain experience they need doing these exams. If money is available to pay patients, it usually provides a superior learning experience.

Use of computer-assisted learning

Many academic settings, especially those with a medical school, have access to computer-assisted instruction. Several programs, notably those developed by Ohio State University through the Health

Education Network, or the Plato Users Network, offer whole courses which serve both as remedial science material or enrichment content. In addition, many computers can be linked through Health Education Network into the Massachusetts General Catalogue which has several case studies developed by Harvard Medical School in which the student analyzes and solves the patients' problems. Many of these case studies are very sophisticated, showing ECG tracings or histological slides. The general technique is to present a patient with a chief complaint, and then the student is allowed to select questions he would ask the computer about the patient. As the student ascertains components of the history, physical examination, and the laboratory work, he constructs a differential diagnosis and treatment modalities. The students win points for how quickly they can arrive at the proper diagnosis, and lose points for arriving at the diagnosis in an incorrect manner. The computer informs them on their progress as they go along, including whether they kill or cure the patient!

Video-taping student interactions with clients

Early in the program it is very useful for students to be video-taped interviewing someone. As the tape is played back it allows them to analyze their own performance as the interviewer. An objective tool should be available to help them evaluate what they do wrong. Tools should specify things such as whether the student asks open-ended questions, interrupts the patient, looks at the patient, writes all the time, talks more than the patient, or uses annoying mannerisms. An extension of this learning technique could be used by having the students video-tape each other as they are learning to examine each body system. Viewing their own examinations, as well as viewing other students examinations, are direct learning experiences.

Video-taping can be used later in the program to actually grade students (i.e., a final examination). Again, this is important if the examination is based on objective criteria. Video-tapes can also be used for research purposes, or to collect data for a variety of purposes in the program. As time goes by students can look at their early films to see how far they have actually progressed.

Sometimes a student might make a video-tape of a patient

encounter. The same tape might be used as a case study, to assess the physical examination, as a self or peer audit, to determine the adequacy of a written note, or to develop a teaching plan. Thus multiple assignments can be built on this single activity.

As students prepare for graduation, video-tape sessions are also helpful as they role-play job interviews. The tapes can then be analyzed to see how they perform, and what they might improve in preparing for an actual interview.

Role-playing

Teachers might rely heavily on the techniques of role-playing, especially in the early phases of the program. Students seem to have an intense need to see faculty members doing the things they want students to do. It is also an excellent opportunity for beginning role-modeling. For example, one instructor might play a patient, another instructor an interviewer. They might demonstrate how a good or bad history should be obtained. During the role play, the faculty can stop to ask students "What type of question should come next?" or "What information should be pursued now?" or "What did we do wrong?" Students can be given a chance to participate by giving suggestions.

Students can also participate in role-playing, and can learn some interviewing techniques by being the patient. What sort of questions are asked that do not get at the information that they want to give? What things do others do that are helpful, or not helpful? This also helps in developing the idea of peer review.

Role-playing can also be a way of presenting case material, in order to liven up presentations, and make content seem more relevant. Faculty or students can act out the drama in the patient encounter.

"Focusing" students in a clinical experience

It may happen that at times there may not be sufficient patients in a clinical setting, necessitating that two students be assigned to care for one patient. The experience might be increased in value by having one student interview and examine the patient, and having the second student "focus" upon the evaluation of the student's performance according to predetermined criteria: comprehensiveness, integration of components of the examination, communication skills, rapport, speed, accuracy, and so on. The notion of peer review is introduced. Each student might write up the history of the patient, and compare the results. How does each student listen?

Criterion-referenced evaluation is often helpful when faculty or students are evaluating the performance of another student. Criterion-referenced evaluation rests upon the development of discrete, observable, objective behaviors or "critical elements" (Lenburg, 1976) which can be seen and measured. These critical elements are in fact mandatory items which the student must do in performing a specified component of the examination. The student knows in the beginning what the critical elements are, and knows they will be expected to demonstrate mastery of these items. Usually 100 percent accuracy of designated items is required.

For example, critical elements pertaining to an examination of the respiratory system might include:

1. Palpates extent of respiratory excursion by placing hands on back at inferior border of the rib cage with thumbs proximal to spinal column.
2. Palpates posterior chest wall for vocal fremitus comparing lung fields.
3. Percusses posterior chest wall bilaterally using mediate percussion technique, moving from side to side comparing each lung field against matching bilateral lung fields.
4. Auscultates breath sounds over each lobe of the lungs, moving stethoscope systematically from side to side and top to bottom, over anterior and lateral surfaces, as well as posterior chest. (Edmunds, Rapson, Singleton, & Steele, 1982).

Requiring the student to perform the specified critical elements allows the faculty to easily and clearly evaluate whether or not the student has performed according to the predetermined standard. Developing criteria that all faculty can agree upon is difficult, but is a strength for a curriculum if it can be done.

Audit activities

Audit involves the notion of looking at performance (of self or others) and judging its adequacy according to defined standards. Nurse practitioners need to learn to look at themselves and others accurately. This is hard to do, and hard to teach students to do. Because nurse practitioners are new in the health care field they are in competition with both more traditional and other new health providers and need to feel comfortable having other people watch, evaluate, and critique them. Audit and quality assurance programs are mandated if nurses plan to receive third party reimbursement. So it is an important technique to develop.

Early in the nurse practitioner program, students need to look at their own clinical performance and their recording of information for evaluative purposes. Thus they must have criteria to evaluate themselves by, or must know how to develop criteria. Forms can be developed for auditing a complete data base, an episodic note, or performance on a component of the physical examination. Use of criterion-referenced tools are often helpful in developing criteria.

Even more difficult to teach than self-audit is the notion of peer review. Students want to stand together and support each other. They feel evaluation often means criticism, and students uniformly do *not* want to criticize each other. But despite these natural tendencies, nurse practitioners need to be able to develop this ability. If nurse practitioners can't or won't evaluate other nurse practitioners, who will evaluate them for the purposes of determining adequacy of their work, reward, or merit? Will this task continue to be left to physicians or other nurse administrative personnel?

In teaching peer audit, begin early in the program. Analyze records anonymously at first. Grade the student who is auditing and not the person being audited. The key to success is to put the burden on the auditor to do a good job. Have both faculty and students audit the same form so interrater reliability can be a goal. Include audit activities in each phase of the program. By the final part of the program, students should be able to audit each other according to defined criteria, and to identify both strong and weak points of performance or write-ups.

STRATEGIES TO KEEP
STUDENTS AND FACULTY AWAKE

The purpose of these special techniques is to provide unusual experiences or activities which will clarify difficult concepts, or provide familiar material in a new manner.

Sometimes a concept is so important that it must be presented several times during the curriculum, each time in a different manner. The repetition helps ensure that students do understand and can apply the material. Such an example might be in teaching about diabetes. Following a lecture, students could follow an ADA diet for a month or two. This experience could lead to development of a lesson plan or teaching script in which the student demonstrates what they have learned which might be helpful to diabetic patients.

One instructor despaired of teaching yet another group of nurse practitioners about myocardial infarction. (This seems to be one content area which must be covered but in which many nurses already feel comfortable, or may have had additional experience.) So the instructor assigned to the class some readings, and on the day of the scheduled lecture, came to class dressed as an old man complaining of chest pain. "He" said he was disillusioned with the young interns in the emergency room, and wanted to talk to someone who might answer his questions about what was happening to him. He then required the students to use their knowledge about heart disease in establishing a differential diagnosis and in determining what should be done. This was a dramatic way of getting students to use information they already had, but putting the responsibility upon them in a way in which they had not experienced it.

Sometimes a point is important enough to go to extra lengths to make sure students remember it. Faculty drama might be another way of creating a lasting impression.

One instructor had emphasized over and over again how it is natural to listen selectively in taking the patient history, often distorting information, or biasing it because of our own personal experiences or beliefs. During the next class period, the instructor staged a quarrel with another instructor. The class lecture was interrupted as the second instructor came into the room, began yelling and complaining, and eventually hit the first instructor. After the second instructor left the room, the first instructor casually asked the group to write down the dialogue that had just taken place, describe the participants, and analyze what was going on. This was followed by listening to the conflicting descriptions and analysis that followed, and then relating it to the main idea of selective listening.

Game playing is another mechanism which could be used periodically to review material which is familiar, or in preparation for an examination. Although many games might be devised, the decision to use a game must be consistent with the objectives of that particular experience. Students should have read extensively on the subject and have had some experience, otherwise game playing is likely to become artificial and pursued largely on the basis of hunches or intuition rather than true knowledge (Bloomfield & Padelford, 1959).

A card game might be developed through construction of a deck of cards relating to a particular disease. One suit of cards would relate to a possible diagnosis, another to treatment, a third to physical findings, another to laboratory values or nonprescription treatments or complications. By drawing, bidding, or trading, students must obtain a card from each category to build a logical case including diagnosis and management. For example, the game might by "Hypertension." A student might have a "Pheochromocytoma" diagnosis card, a physical examination card indicating "sweating, flushing, paroxysmal tachycardia, spontaneous elevations in blood pressure" and a treatment card indicating "surgery." (This same technique could be used for a variety of diseases: lung disease, anemias, kidney tract infections, etc.)

Board games might also be developed which allow students to move a certain number of squares based upon answers they give to questions which are printed on prepared cards. Certain spaces on the board have traps, or complications, which require the student to fall back spaces. Other spaces on the board allow the student to have remissions, or cures, or they don't have to pay their hospital bills, and allow them to move forward. The number of spaces the student can advance is determined by the card. Whether the student answers correctly is determined by the group.

A number of commercially available games is already on the

market and might be purchased for use. There are also a growing number of nursing publications describing games which can be used (Wolf & Duffy, 1979).

Active games can also be developed, allowing the students to move forward or backward (much like the board games) based on their answers to questions. Patterns of movement can be drawn on the floor with chalk, and teams can be formed to answer and direct movement of players.

Sometimes using games or role-playing is not enough. It may be necessary for the student to actually experience what is being discussed. For example, having a nasogastric tube, wearing a nasal cannula, and having a rectal exam can all be personal learning events. Going through the experience is much more advantageous than having someone tell you about what is involved. Whenever students can be involved and actually do the thing being discussed, the learning will be superior.

SUMMARY

In attempting to evaluate the numerous techniques which might be used to strengthen a curriculum, many factors must be taken into account. Sometimes listing all the possible strategies and evaluating them along various parameters help determine which things are worth spending time and money to include in the curriculum.

The evaluation tool in Figure 9-1 is suggested as one way of examining some of the techniques suggested in this chapter for inclusion in a curriculum. Across the left-hand side of the page are five major parameters which might be important to rate techniques against. Across the right top of the page, list the possible strategies which might be used. Evaluate each strategy in turn, marking each category with a plus (+) if a technique seems desirable and reasonable, a minus (−) if it would not be possible, or is unappealing, and a question mark (?) if it is unclear whether this would be practical or not. A grouping of (+) marks should indicate where time and money should be devoted in developing innovative teaching strategies for your program (see Figure 9-1).

STRATEGIES
(Techniques or Assignments)

PARAMETERS												
1. Resources available for using strategies												
a. fiscal												
b. faculty interest												
c. student creativity												
d. equipment												
e. other												
2. Time for development of methodologies												
a. early in curriculum development												
b. later in curriculum												
3. Complexity of strategies chosen												
4. Need for innovative strategies												
a. to present content												
b. reinforce important material												
c. fill in gaps in existing curriculum												
d. other												
5. Desirability of this strategy in adding variety to present program												

Figure 9-1. Parameters for Evaluating Possible Teaching Strategies

Use of new and creative teaching strategies has several long-term benefits:

Student benefits

- increased content retention
- content made more meaningful
- program seems "alive"
- enthusiasm develops
- quantity and quality of planning and preparation of faculty are visible

Teacher benefits

- opportunity to teach content which must be repeated year after year in a variety of ways
- different teaching methods can be tried with varying classes to see which forms have the most benefit
- assists teacher in staying up to date, prepared
- aids in presenting material effectively
- wisely utilizes class and clinical time

Curriculum benefits

- constant and careful scrutiny of ideas in order to determine what should be taught, sequencing, and how content and experiences reinforce each other. Because of this, use of innovative strategies may be a strength to the curriculum.
- infusion of new ideas which come from faculty and student exchange makes the curriculum vibrant.
- the curriculum is imbued with additional creative efforts of many contributors.

REFERENCES

Bloomfield, L. P. & Padelford, N. J. Three experiments in political gaming. *American Political Science Review*, 1959, *53*, 1105–1115.

Bridgman, C. F. & Suter, E. Searching AVLINE for curriculum related audiovisual instructional material. *Journal of Medical Education*, 1979, *54*, 236–337.

Dale, E. (Ed.). *Audiovisual methods in teaching*. Hillsdale, Illinois: The Dryden Press, 1969.

Edmunds, M. W. Conflict. *The Nurse Practitioner*, 1979, *4* (6), 42, 47–48.

Edmunds, M. W. Developing a marketing portfolio. *The Nurse Practitioner*, 1980, *5* (3), 41–46.

Edmunds, M. W., Rapson, M., Singleton, E., & Steele, S. Development of a criterion-referenced evaluation tool to measure health assessment skills of graduate students. Manuscript submitted for publication, 1982.

Hudak, C. M., Redstone, P. M., Hokanson, N. L., & Suzuki, I. E. *Clinical protocols: A guide for nurses and physicians*. Philadelphia: J. B. Lippincott Company, 1976, 4–5.

Lenburg, C. *Criteria for developing clinical performance evaluation*. National League for Nursing, 1976, 1–16. Pub. No. 23–1634.

Maatsch, J. L. A study of simulation technology in medical education: Main paper, mimeographed (East Lansing, Michigan: Office of Medical Education, Research Development, Michigan State University, 1978, p. 10) quoted in M. W. Wolf & M. E. Duffy, *Simulations/games: A teaching strategy for nursing education*. National League for Nursing, 1979, 18. Pub. No. 23–1756.

Russell, J. D. *Modular instruction: A guide to the design, selection, utilization, and policy evaluation of modular materials*. Minneapolis, Minnesota: Burgess, 1974.

Wolf, M. S. & Duffy, M. E. *Simulations/games: A teaching strategy for nursing education*. National League for Nursing, 1979, Pub. No. 23–1756.

III
Evaluation and Research

10

Program Evaluation

Nurse educators have been accused of being preoccupied with evaluation—of spending more time evaluating than implementing programs. Certainly there is great interest in the evaluation of expanded-role programs. Of primary concern is the competence of graduates in new roles. Many studies—few done by nurses, unfortunately—have compared nurse practitioner students and graduates to medical students, physicians, physicians' assistants, and nurses in traditional roles in personal attributes, competencies, and practice preferences (Edmunds, 1978; Prescott & Driscoll, 1979). These are important aspects of program evaluation but not the total picture. Total program evaluation is a comprehensive plan to examine many facets.

THE EVALUATION PROCESS

Educational evaluation is defined as the process used in determining the effectiveness of teaching and/or the value of a learning opportunity in assisting students to meet program objectives (Conley, 1973, p. 342). A comprehensive evaluation should be based on some rational conceptual view of the educational program. A commonly used framework is based on general systems theory where the educational program (i.e., course, degree-granting program, continuing education program) can be seen as having inputs, processes or operations, and outputs (Astin & Panos, 1971; Staropoli & Waltz, 1978). These elements will vary with the program, but the principle is that various inputs into the program interact through designated processes or operations to produce outputs. In an educational system, one desired output is a graduate who has met the predetermined objectives of the course or program. In its simplest form the equation is:

$$
\begin{array}{ccc}
\text{STUDENTS AND} & + \text{ TEACHING-} & = & \text{STUDENTS} \\
\text{TEACHERS} & \text{LEARNING} & & \text{WITH NEW} \\
 & & & \text{COMPETENCIES} \\
\text{(Inputs)} & \text{(Process)} & & \text{(Output)}
\end{array}
$$

However, in modern education, all three segments are much more complex than the skeleton equation indicates. In most nursing programs the inputs will include:

1. Students
    a. demographic characteristics
    b. academic, personal, and personality characteristics
    c. skill level in nursing or prerequisite knowledge
    d. motivation and aspirations
2. Faculty
    a. experience in nursing and teaching
    b. academic qualifications
    c. personal and personality characteristics
3. Other resources
    a. money
    b. time
    c. space
    d. texts, audiovisual software, other equipment

Examples of processes found in a nursing program are:

1. Teaching
    a. instructional methods
    b. content
2. Environment-student interaction

3. Student-student interaction
4. Student-patient interaction
5. Student-health professional interaction

Typical outputs are:

1. New skills and competencies (learning)
2. A greater number of qualified practitioners
3. Teacher and learner satisfaction
4. Cost of program

These are only a few of the inputs, processes, and outputs expected in a nursing education program. Those that are most central to the teaching process should be included in an evaluation.

Assumptions

Several assumptions are inherent in the evaluation process:

1. All domains of learning can be appraised by some method.
2. Evaluation of a sample can be generalized (i.e., student's clinical competence, the learning environment, or the faculty's teaching).
3. There is a relationship between the inputs, processes, and outcomes of an educational program.

If these can be accepted, an evaluation effort is worthwhile and, indeed, necessary to improve the program.

Scope

It is impossible to identify and evaluate all possible inputs, processes, and outputs that may have an impact. The scope of an evaluation plan usually is determined pragmatically by the amount of resources that can be committed. One method of determining the scope is to prepare an overall plan, then select and prioritize those areas that will have the greatest yield. For instance, determining the cost per student may be a first priority if a department or school budget is in preparation, whereas an analysis of the learning environment or admissions requirements may be very important if the student drop-out rate is high.

To prepare a comprehensive evaluation plan, there are five major questions to answer:

1. Why is the evaluation being conducted?
2. Who is to be involved?
3. What is to be evaluated?
4. When should it take place?
5. How is the program to be evaluated?

This framework was proposed by Holzemer in Staropoli and Waltz (1978, pp. 88–108) and is used as a basis for the organization of this chapter.

CHOOSING THE EVALUATORS

Several categories of people who are affected by the results of an expanded-role program evaluation should be involved. They may be either participants in the formulation of the evaluation plan, a source of data, or both. For instance, teachers may help construct an evaluation plan and, in turn, be evaluated.

Planners

Those who plan educational programs such as school administrators, faculty, and funding sources are potential audiences for evaluation results. They should have the opportunity to identify the data they need for decision making.

Participants

Graduates, students, and potential students are also audiences as well as data sources. Applicants are interested in how well an existing program meets its stated objectives. Current students want to know, among other things, where their performance stands in relation to other students and in relation to what they will need on completion.

Faculty are participants as well as planners. Their interest may be in several areas of evaluation such as student progress, teacher effectiveness, effect of the learning environment, and employment history of graduates.

Employers

Actual and potential employers of nurse practitioners are sources of data and an audience for results. They are interested in what is taught and the level of competence of graduates. In turn, they can indicate the need for and acceptance of a nurse practitioner.

The public

Several segments of the public are concerned with the outcomes of evaluation. Potential clients want to know how well a professional such as a nurse practitioner can provide for their health needs. Others may be concerned about the cost of education, cost of services, or the general economic impact of nurse practitioners.

The evaluators

Finally, the discussion must be made about who will be directly involved in the evaluation. Usually, a committee is formed to construct the evaluation plan and to implement it. The membership depends on the organizational structure of the school and the scope of the evaluation. A comprehensive evaluation of a new master's program preparing family nurse practitioners might include the administrator of the program, one or more higher-level administrators, and faculty representatives. Evaluation experts on the faculty can be committee members or consultants. Similarly, outside experts can be used to formulate the plan or to offer consultation throughout the implementation and evaluation of the plan.

If only a course or a continuing education offering is being evaluated or a specific segment of a program, representative evaluators are chosen, although it may be wise to have other disinterested parties involved. A program or course evaluation should fit into any existing overall school evaluation plan. Efforts should be made to use available expertise, and to be efficient as well as effective in producing usable results.

PURPOSES OF EVALUATION

The first task of the evaluator or committee is to clarify the "why" for an evaluation. Most nursing programs or courses are evaluated for one of the following reasons:

1. Determine if program objectives are being met.
2. Identify needs for curriculum revision (including revision of objectives and purposes of the program).
3. Determine if a program meets the needs of the public and the health care delivery system.
4. Assess personal and personality characteristics of applicants or new students.
5. Assess beginning or ongoing competencies of students.
6. Analyze the factors affecting student learning (i.e., clinical placements, instructional methods, supervision).
7. Improve instruction.
8. Determine teacher effectiveness.
9. Determine placement and job characteristics of graduates.
10. Provide data for informing the public of the success of a program.
11. Report the status of a program to a potential or actual funding source (Conley, 1973; Staropoli & Waltz, 1978).

SCOPE OF EVALUATION

It is evident that the purposes listed above are met by evaluating inputs, processes, outcomes, or a combination of two or more of these. Inherent in each purpose are questions that can be asked. For a program preparing adult nurse practitioners, typical questions are given in the following examples:

Example A

Purpose: to assess beginning competencies of students
Possible questions:

1. At what level can beginning students perform a total health assessment?
2. What are the communication skills of beginning students?
3. What knowledge of pathophysiology do beginning students have?

Example B

Purpose: to improve instruction
Possible questions:

1. What combination of clinical experience and theoretical knowledge is needed to prepare a competent nurse practitioner?
2. What content is best taught by nursing versus non-nursing faculty?
3. What instructional method is best for teaching the identification of normal heart sounds?

Example C

Purpose: to report the status of a program to the funding agency
Possible questions:

1. How many students have (a) been admitted; (b) dropped out; (c) completed the program?
2. Who participated in teaching the students?
3. How were students evaluated?

It is apparent that the complexity of questions posed for evaluation can vary depending on the scope of the purposes. When the purposes of an evaluation are determined an exhaustive list of questions can be developed with subordinate questions where necessary. Then the scope and depth of the effort can be determined based on needs and available resources. It may be necessary to prioritize and stage the evaluation effort over several months or years. For instance, determining entrance characteristics is a cumulative process and may require several classes to give an accurate picture of applicants. On the other hand, testing of instructional methods can be ongoing.

Describing the program

To provide background for the evaluators and the potential audiences, a description of the program is necessary. Generally this includes identification of the inputs, processes, and outcomes of the program. At the least, this preliminary effort should describe the participants in the program, what happens to them, and the product. This exercise may reveal additional purposes and questions for the evaluation and also may point out what data are not available (Staropoli & Waltz, 1978, pp. 93–94).

Timing of the evaluation

The points at which evaluation should occur depend primarily on *what* is evaluated and on the resources available. Beginning characteristics of students must be measured prior to or within a few days after entrance or the data may be contaminated by the effects of the program. Similarly, the chronological proximity of two events can affect results. For example, asking students to evaluate teachers immediately after a difficult examination may produce different results than if the two events are not time-related.

Most program evaluations are a combination of *formative* and *summative* methods. Formative evaluation is that which occurs throughout the program and involves inputs and processes. Summative evaluation is concerned with the outcomes of an educational experience. Usually it focuses on student outcomes but may also measure costs, impact on health care delivery, patients, public, or employers.

The value of formative evaluation is that immediate feedback can be used to correct deficiencies and improve the program. However, some caution is advised in making frequent modifications based on insufficient data. There is danger that cause and effect relationships will be assumed where none exist. This is particularly true of the evaluation of teaching strategies. Because learning is a complex process, the changing of one element may not improve the outcome. For example, the inability of the majority of students in a class to demonstrate a knowledge of the symptoms of congestive heart failure may not be the result of a poor lecture but for one or more diverse reasons such as an inadequate background in physiology, inappropriate sequencing of content, a poor classroom environment, or failure to study because of anxiety after a classmate's automobile accident.

The purpose of formative evaluation should be clearly determined and the timing carefully chosen. Usually data are needed for giving grades at the end of each course so that testing of theoretical knowledge will occur then. Teacher retention, merit, and promotion decisions are made yearly so that teacher effectiveness can be summarized then, even though data may be collected at several times. Practicality and utility should dictate the type and frequency of formative evaluation.

Summative evaluation, by definition, occurs at the end of a program. However, data on graduates should be collected at defined periods after completion such as six months, one year, or five years. This is especially important in a nurse practitioner program where a new type of practitioner is being prepared. Role and job characteristics including graduate, patient, and employer satisfaction are important information to feed back to the program planners.

Another type of evaluation, *comparative*, is also appropriate for a nurse practitioner program. Here one program is compared to another. There is great interest in how nurse practitioner students and graduates compare to other health professional students, other nurses, and graduates of other nurse practitioner programs. These comparisons can be made on characteristics of students, interim and terminal competencies, or on employment sites, tasks, and roles assumed.

METHODS OF EVALUATION

A variety of methods can be used to answer the predetermined questions for evaluation. For example, the assessment of competencies of beginning students may be measured by a paper and pencil achievement test or by observation of clinical skills. The attitudes of the public or patients about nurse practitioners can be surveyed by an open-ended or forced-choice questionnaire administered by phone, mail, or in person. Choosing the proper methods and instruments is critical. Otherwise the results may be meaningless.

Instruments

Evaluation methods chosen should have the following characteristics:

1. *Reliability* is the accuracy (consistency and stability) of measurement by an instrument. This may be determined by retesting after a period of time, by calculating a measure of internal consistency (i.e., alpha), by using parallel forms, or by calculating intra- and interrater reliability for observer measures.
2. *Validity* is the degree to which a test measures what it purports to measure. Content validity is demonstrated by showing how well items sample the construct to be measured. Criterion-related validity is estimated by comparing the results of one measure to that of another criterion. One form, predictive validity, refers to the extent that future scores are predicted by a prior measure. The other, concurrent validity, refers to the agreement of results on two measures used at the same time. The reader is referred to Gronlund (1968), Staropoli and Waltz (1978), or texts on measurement and evaluation for a more detailed discussion of reliability and validity.
3. *Practicality* dictates that an instrument must be affordable and efficient in terms of time, effort, and expense. For example, the test administrator should not require extensive training. A measure should not collect a large amount of extraneous data.

Most nursing education programs are evaluated using one or more of the following methods for collecting data:

- *Observation:* The process of observing conditions or activities. The data collected are descriptive, such as an anecdotal record, or quantitative, as in a rating scale.
- *Standardized test:* An objective test for which norms have been established, uniform methods of administering and scoring have been developed, and content validated. Ex-

amples are the state board examination for nurses or the certification examinations for nurse practitioners.

- *Teacher-made test:* Created by one individual or group for local use.
- *Essay test:* The student is asked to discuss, enumerate, evaluate, or otherwise demonstrate a degree of understanding of a topic in a properly written composition.
- *Objective test:* A test constructed so that independent evaluators will award the same score for a given performance. These are usually multiple-choice, matching, or completion although some observational measures can be somewhat objective. The degree of objectivity is measured by calculating interrater reliability.
- *Achievement test:* A test that measures a person's knowledge, skills, and understanding of a given content.
- *Diagnostic test:* A test that permits the identification of strengths and weaknesses in a given area. It can be a written or performance test.
- *Inventory:* A listing of objects, defined characteristics, interests, abilities, or preferences. Equipment and other environmental characteristics can be inventoried as can student, faculty, or employer characteristics.
- *Questionnaire:* A list of questions on a particular topic with space for one or more forced-choice responses.
- *Rating scale:* A method used in assessing characteristics on an ordinal scale. (Conley, 1973)

This list is not exhaustive or its components mutually exclusive. Other methods and instruments may be appropriate for a given evaluation. Evaluators must choose the most reliable, valid, and practical methods to answer the questions selected. Consultants are often knowledgeable about preexisting instruments so that faculty do not have to spend valuable resources developing their own. Where this is necessary, instruments should be pretested and their reliability and validity determined.

Table 10-1 lists some typical methods for evaluating some elements of a nurse practitioner program. The reader is also referred

Table 10-1. Evaluation Methods for Selected Program Elements

ELEMENT	METHODS, DATA SOURCES
(I)* <u>Students</u>	
Attitudes	Rating scales; anecdotal records; questionnaires.
Achievement	Observation; objective tests; essay tests; oral examination; simulations.
(I) <u>Faculty</u>	
Academic qualifications	Curriculum vitae; questionnaires.
Competency	Questionnaires from peers, students, supervisors; observation; student achievement; research and publication products.
(P)* <u>Teaching strategies</u>	Observation; student achievement; costs in time, money, effort.
(P) <u>Student role change</u>	Essays; observation; rating scales – several times during program.
(O)* <u>Student competencies</u>	Achievement at end of program; final clinical examination; certification exams.
(O) <u>Employer satisfaction</u>	Survey, observation, telephone interviews.
(O) <u>Impact of graduates</u>	Surveys of employers for change in practice patterns and economic impact; patient surveys or interviews; alumni surveys.

<u>*Key</u>

I = Input   P = Process   O = Output

to Booth (1978) for a proposed plan for evaluating a master's nurse practitioner program.

EVALUATION OF STUDENT COMPETENCE

The concern over the quality of care and safe practice of nurses in expanded roles has led to a concerted effort in developing instruments to measure clinical competence. Some of the issues are not unique to the expanded role. Evaluators ask:

1. What should be measured to ensure clinical competence?
2. Who should have input into clinical evaluation?
3. How can the reliability and validity of measures of clinical performance be improved?
4. How can clinical performance be sampled reliably?
5. What is the role of written tests in assessing clinical competence?

Because evaluation of students and graduates in expanded roles is not covered comprehensively in other literature and because it is controversial and has far-reaching effects, this aspect of evaluation deserves added attention. The testing of theoretical knowledge alone is covered in many other sources. Teachers of nurse practitioners use the same principles in developing multiple-choice, essay, and other written tests as teachers in other fields. The reader is referred to several sources listed at the end of the chapter for techniques in test construction for cognitive knowledge. The emphasis here is on the application of that knowledge to the clinical setting.

Clinical competence involves the application of cognitive, psychomotor, and affective learning. Knowledge from many sources is needed to provide primary care to sick and well individuals. Much of this is tested in prerequisite courses such as anatomy, pharmacology, psychology. It is practical to test only learning that should occur as a result of current courses. For example, in a course for pediatric nurse practitioners on the well child, this includes learning such as the proper immunization schedule for infants. Testing for this knowledge will occur in some type of written examination or in a programmed learning sequence. However, the ultimate test is whether or not the student checks the immunization record of each infant seen in a real clinical setting. This can only be ascertained by audit of records or reporting to a preceptor.

Direct observation methods

Most schools have developed their own forms for rating students based on the SOAP or the traditional medical history and physical formats. Appendix 2 is a brief tool that can be used for audit of peer or self. It is only appropriate when a new problem is identified. It could be modified for health promotion or screening visits.

Appendix 3 is a form for evaluating a student at the end of a course in the management of children's health care. Note that there is a section requiring validation by the instructor. The accuracy of the history can be validated by asking the parent or child a few selected questions or reviewing tape or video recordings. Repeating history questions must be done with care because too much repetition will decrease both the student's and patient's confidence. However, to assure safe and higher-quality care, errors in diagnosis must be corrected tactfully. Appendix 4 is a general form for clinical evaluation but is most appropriate with adult patients.

Other formats for collecting and recording observations of clinical practice are available. The Nurse Practitioner Rating Form was used in several research studies where the reliability was checked (Goodwin, Prescott, Jacox & Collar, 1981). This instrument measures the frequency of several activity categories: history-taking; physical examination; treatment and procedures; advice, directions, or instructions; facts; explanations; demonstrations; and consultation. The content in each category is further classified to differentiate psychosocial and physiological aspects of care.

Simulations

It is not always possible to find patients with conditions or needs that students should learn to manage. Many of the creative methods in Chapter 9 can be standardized and used for testing as well as teaching. This includes role playing, professional patients, computer case simulation, and written clinical simulations. McLaughlin (1978) developed two written case simulations for patients with COPD and hypertension. These are very common problems so that these well-developed written simulations can be used for testing adult or family nurse practitioners. Some simulations have been developed for medical students and physicians and are usually known as PMPs (Patient Management Problems). They can also be used if they are modified to include nursing care.

Criterion-referenced tests

The typical test used in evaluating students is norm-referenced. This type compares students with one another by awarding grades on a continuum. It is an excellent method for selecting the students with the best performance. However, the wisdom of norm-referenced testing in measuring safe and competent practice has been questioned. Competency-based or criterion-referenced testing is an alternative. In this method, desired behaviors are delineated in detail with as much accuracy as possible. The student is then graded only as to whether or not the criterion is met. If the test is written, a percentage of items that must be passed is predetermined. The same can be done with psychomotor skills. For instance, three items on a health assessment examination might be:

1. Assesses full active and passive range of motion of all major joints.
2. Assesses cerebellar function using two maneuvers.
3. Elicits health history of siblings, parents, and grandparents.

The student would either perform the given task in total as written or would not pass that item.

Some benefits of criterion-referenced tests are that they:

1. Can be used for self-paced instruction.
2. Can be used for student guidance.
3. Assure that critical behaviors are learned.

Competency-based assessment should occur at entry, at regular intervals during a program, and at the end of a program or course. Only summative assessments should be used for grading purposes. Earlier assessments are used to counsel students on strengths and weaknesses and to plan additional learning experiences. Six essential characteristics criterion-referenced tests must have are:

1. An explicit description of the competency to be measured.
2. Sufficient number of measures per assessed competency.
3. Sufficiently limited focus.
4. Assurance of reliable results (are repeatable).
5. Assurance of validity.
6. Availability of comparative data on other students.

Competency-based measurement is not the panacea for all the problems of norm-referenced testing but psychometricians and educators have addressed many of the concerns. (See van der Linden, 1982, for a review.) Some of these are the optimum length of a test, item analysis, and choosing of a cut-off score. Thus far it appears to be a good method of assuring competencies in clinical practice.

Assessing affective learning

Provided that affective objectives are included in student's expectations, they must be assessed. These include attitudes, values, and biases that are expressed verbally, in writing, or through nonverbal actions. Because the instructor's own values are involved, measuring of students' affective behavior must be done with care and fairness. Particularly important are those behaviors concerned with taking on an expanded role. A student who asks many questions and expresses doubts may be developing a more positive attitude than the student who indicates no problem taking on the role. It may be necessary to give a written assignment or ask for a reaction to a situation to elicit data for evaluating affective learning. Other important areas for which objectives should be developed and evaluated are in attitudes about cultural differences, confidentiality, informed consent, mutuality of nurse-patient goals, and interprofessional practice.

Multiple measures

The evaluation of clinical competence in students or graduates is complex. Emphasis in nurse practitioner programs to date has been on technical performance, perhaps because it is new learning to be integrated into a base of nursing knowledge. However, the role has matured enough that competence in total patient care should be measured. For instance, a complete data base and initial plan should include psychosocial competencies as well as physical problems and in the same depth. To measure such competencies, new instruments must be developed or old ones modified to include all aspects of nurse practitioner practice.

Since they lack standardized measures that are valid and reliable, instructors would do well to use several methods to measure clinical competence. A paper and pencil multiple-choice test, a patient management problem, a computer-assisted test, simulations, or direct observation can be used to test knowledge and competence in patient care. Input from direct observation of a physician preceptor should be valued, but the responsibility for student evaluation remains with the nurse faculty. Peers can be of benefit in auditing records and observing performance, but they should not be responsible for summative evaluation.

Not only should multiple measures of clinical competence be used but, within practicality, they should be given at intervals for both formative and summative purposes. Mechanisms for feedback to students must be established so that students and instructors together can work to upgrade deficiencies. Praise and validation, judiciously used, can instill the self-confidence needed in a new role.

IMPLEMENTATION OF THE PLAN

When the purposes (why), questions (what), appropriate methods (how), and timing (when) are determined, the evaluation committee or a selected evaluator implements the plan. Adjustments may be needed as data are collected. Additions or changes are made if a vital area has been overlooked or a method is inappropriate. There must be ongoing evaluation of the evaluation plan too. Is it doing what was expected? Is it practical and efficient? If not, changes must be made.

As data are compiled and analyzed, written reports should be given to the various audiences. Process evaluation may indicate an immediate need for change. Sequencing of content, guest lecturers, and student testing are areas that can be modified rather quickly given valid and reliable information. Other measures are longer term such as the number of graduates who are working in various settings and their satisfaction with the role.

Setting criteria

Inevitably, an evaluator or committee must use the data collected to answer the evaluation questions. If the question involves a determination of quality or adequacy of performance, a consensus is necessary. Often the criteria are internal but, nonetheless, influence the decisions. It is preferable to come to consensus on such criteria as passing grades on examinations, teacher-student ratios, and percentage of admitted students that should complete the program successfully. Other judgments will admittedly be less clear and may require external consultation to set a criterion. For example, the decision as to whether a program is cost-effective may require comparison with other departments and schools and the consultation of a costing expert.

PROGRAM REVISION

Evaluation efforts are wasted if there is no response to the feedback from the evaluation effort. Conversely, curriculum change without solid data indicating a need is wasteful. Any program that is thoughtfully designed and executed deserves to run through at least one cycle without major revision. Yet where change is urgently indicated, equally thoughtful plans to improve the program should be undertaken. Some of the typical program areas in nurse practitioner programs that undergo change are admission requirements, qualification of faculty, clinical placements, and criteria for clinical competence. These cause the most concern because they are the areas that differ the most from other nursing programs.

Resistance to change

Nurse educators who plan and develop expanded-role programs have been pioneers in many ways. Much of their professional identity is vested in the program they create, so that when change is suggested either by an internal committee or outside consultant, it may be resisted. It means the expenditure of more time and energy to develop alternatives to the problem area. In addition, territoriality may play a part. It is difficult to discard, change, or share content or methods that represent faculty's own creativity and "belongs" to them.

Other changes may be due to a decrease or increase in funding, or direction from higher administration. Competition for students may instigate a new track or emphasis area so that the program is more marketable. A change in society's need for certain types of nurses is another reason for program revision.

In the past few years, a great deal of literature has been devoted to the planning of change. Before curriculum revision is undertaken, the reader would benefit from becoming knowledgeable with some techniques in the planning and managing of change (i.e., Bennis, Benne & Chinn, 1976). One of the prime considerations is to be aware that a change in one part of a system may cause a disequilibrium in another. Evaluators must consider the "ripple effect" of changing teaching strategies, content, or objectives. Will offering a new track weaken the already successful existing program? If nurse faculty teach more of the diagnosis and management content, will they deemphasize the nursing component?

REEVALUATION

Finally, the evaluation process comes full circle. The changes are implemented and are, in turn, evaluated. Some schools find it profitable to have a continuous evaluation cycle with certain parts scheduled at regular intervals and others ongoing.

SUMMARY

Program evaluation includes deciding who should participate, why it is being conducted, what is to be evaluated, when it should occur, and how it is to be accomplished. Pertinent questions about the input, processes, and output of the educational program are posed and methods chosen to answer them. Data are collected and the questions answered. When appropriate, criteria for answering the questions are developed. Program changes are made in response to the evaluation effort and are, in turn, evaluated.

REFERENCES

Astin, A. & Panos, R. J. The evaluation of educational programs. In R. L. Thorndike, (Ed.), *Educational Measurement*. 2nd ed. Washington, D.C.: American Council on Education, 1971.

Bennis, W. G., Benne, K. D., & Chinn, R. *The planning of change*, 3rd ed. New York: Holt, Rinehart and Winston, 1976.

Booth, R. Sample evaluation plan. In C. J. Staropoli & C. F. Waltz, *Developing and evaluating educational programs for health care providers*. Philadelphia: F. A. Davis Company, 1978.

Conley, V. C. *Curriculum and instruction in nursing*. Boston: Little, Brown and Company, 1973.

Edmunds, M. W. Evaluation of nurse practitioner effectiveness: An overview of the literature. *Evaluation and the Health Professions*, 1978, *1*, (1), 69–81.

Fitts, P. M. & Posner, M. I. *Human performance*. Belmont, California: Brooks/Cole Publishing Company, 1967.

Goodwin, L. D., Prescott, P., Jacox, A., & Collar, M. The nurse practitioner rating form: Part II. *Nursing Research*, 1981, *30*, 270–276.

Gronlund, N. E. (Ed.). *Readings in measurement and evaluation*. New York: Macmillan, 1968.

McLaughlin, Frank. *Primary care judgments of nurses and physicians* (3 volumes). San Francisco: Veterans Administration Hospital, 1978.

Prescott, P. A. & Driscoll, L. Nurse practitioner effectiveness: A review of physician-nurse practitioner comparison studies. *Evaluation and the Health Professionals*, 1979, 2, (4), 387–418.

Staropoli, C. J. & Waltz, C. F. *Developing and evaluating educational programs for health care providers*. Philadelphia: F. A. Davis Company, 1978.

van der Linden, W. J. Criterion-referenced measurement: Its main application, problems, and findings. *Evaluation in Education*, 1982, 5, 97–118.

SUGGESTED READINGS

Anderson, S. B., Murphy, T., & Associates. *Encyclopedia of educational evaluation*. San Francisco: Jossey-Bass, 1978.

Arney, W. R. Evaluation of a continuing nursing education program and its implications. *The Journal of Continuing Education in Nursing*, 1978, 9, (1), 45–51.

Berk, R. A. (Ed.). *Criterion-referenced measurement: The state of the art.* Baltimore: Johns Hopkins University Press, 1980.

Centra, J. A. *Determining faculty effectiveness.* San Francisco: Jossey-Bass, 1977.

Doyle, K. O. *Student evaluation of instructors.* Lexington, Massachusetts: Lexington Books, 1975.

Ebel, R. L. *Measuring educational achievement.* Englewood Cliffs, New Jersey: Prentice-Hall, 1965.

Forbes, E. & Nelson, T. *The clinical evaluation dilemma: A survey of problems encountered by faculty.* New York: National League for Nursing, 1979.

French, J. W. & Michel, W. B. The nature and meaning of validity and reliability, In E. E. Gronlund (Ed.), *Readings in measurement and evaluation.* New York: Macmillan, 1968.

Frisbie, D. A. *Evaluating student achievement: Principles, trends, and problems.* New York: National League for Nursing, 1979.

Greenlick, M. R. Assessing clinical competence: A societal review. *Evaluation and the Health Professions*, 1981, 4, 3–12.

Gronlund, N. E. *Measurement and evaluation in teaching*, 4th ed. New York: Macmillan, 1981.

Ketefian, S. A paradigm for faculty evaluation. *Nursing Outlook*, 25 (10), 718–720.

Knopke, H. J. & Goodwin, B. B. Assessing student competence. In H. J. Knopke & N. L. Diekelmann (Eds.), *Approaches to teaching primary care.* St. Louis: C. V. Mosby Company, 1981.

Knox, B. (Ed.). *Assessing the impact of continuing education.* San Francisco: Jossey-Bass, 1979.

Krathwohl, D. R., Bloom, B. S., & Masia, B. B. *Taxonomy of educational objectives. Handbook II. The affective domain.* New York: Longmans, Inc., 1969.

Marriner, A., Langford, T., & Goodwin, L. D. Curriculum evaluation: Wordfact, ritual, or reality. *Nursing Outlook*, 1980, 28, (4), 228–232.

McGuire, C. H. & Solomon, L. *Clinical simulations: Selected problems in patient management*, 2nd ed. New York: Appleton-Century-Crofts, 1976.

Morgan, M. K. & Irby, D. M. *Evaluating clinical competence in the health professions.* St. Louis: C. V. Mosby Company, 1978.

National League for Nursing. *Evaluation of teaching effectiveness.* New York: NLN, 1977.

Newble, D. I., Elmslie, R. G., & Baxter, A. A problem-based criterion-referenced examination of clinical competence. *Journal of Medical Education*, 1978, *53*, 720–726.

Popham, W. J. *Evaluation in education*. Berkeley, California: McCutchan Publishing Company, 1974.

Popham, W. J., (Ed.). *Criterion-referenced measurement*. Englewood Cliffs, New Jersey: Prentice-Hall, 1978.

Prescott, P. A., Jacox, A., Collar, M., & Goodwin, L. The nurse practitioner rating form, Part I. *Nursing Research*, 1981, *30*, (4), 223–228.

Reese, J. L., Swanson, A. E., & Cunning, B. R. Evaluating physical assessment skills. *Nursing Outlook*, 1979, *27*, (10), 662–665.

Rossi, P. H. & Freeman, H. E. *Evaluation: A systematic approach*, 2nd ed. Beverly Hills: Sage Publications, 1982.

Schneider, H. L. *Evaluation of nursing competence*. Boston: Little, Brown and Company, 1979.

Thorndike, R. L. (Ed.). *Educational measurement*, 2nd ed. Washington: American Council on Education, 1971.

Tyler, R. W. (Ed.). *Educational evaluation: New roles, new means*. Chicago: University of Chicago Press, 1969.

Weed, L. L. *Medical records, medical education, and patient care: The problem-oriented record as a basic tool*. Cleveland: Case Western Reserve University Press, 1970.

11

Research Opportunities

In the first years of the nurse practitioner movement, the literature was replete with "this I believe" articles. Some interesting debates took place in the pages of nursing journals regarding expanded roles. This was a necessary first step as educators and practitioners gained experience and formulated attitudes.

The next step was the reporting of studies either describing student or graduate characteristics or comparing them to physicians or physicians' assistants in practice patterns and patient management. The results supported the competence of nurse practitioners and, in fact, often failed to emphasize that in some studies they outperformed other health care providers (Prescott & Driscoll, 1980). Many of these studies were undertaken by physicians or professional evaluators rather than nurses and hence failed to include many variables related to nursing practice. Other methodological problems were inherent in these early comparison studies such as considering only functions of the nurse practitioner that were also done by physicians.

The time is ripe for a new generation of research and evaluation studies to be conducted by nurse researchers who are knowledgeable and sophisticated in clinical expertise, teaching, and research methods. Furthermore, the growth and development of expanded roles for nursing in a time of a shrinking economy will be dependent upon accurate data on which schools, governmental bodies, and health care systems can base program decisions. For instance, third party reimbursement for several nursing functions is relatively new in a few states. Extension of this boost to independent practice will be based on the identification of a unique nursing role and a consumer demand for it. In another area, external funders will want to know that the most cost-effective methods of instruction are being used in a proposed program.

There are several very good reasons why teachers of primary care should engage in research and publication. First, their combination of skills and knowledge of primary care teaching and clinical practice is unique in nursing, and there is a responsibility to build knowledge in the field. Second, the increasing demand in academe that nurse faculty meet the same criteria for promotion and tenure as other teachers makes research and publishing a high priority for most university and college-level teachers. Last is the responsibility to find better ways to care for people, both sick and well. Many primary care faculty are completing doctorates or are developing research skills and are now prepared to make a major contribution.

RESEARCH IN EDUCATION

Several general categories of research activities are appropriate for primary care faculty. Some are in the larger category of evaluation research. This differs from the evaluation process described in the last chapter where the only purpose is program evaluation. In evaluation research, evaluation methods that were mentioned in Chapter 10 can be studied using scientific methods and techniques. Of particular interest at this stage of expanded-role development are:

1. Admissions requirements.
2. Predictors of success.
3. Clinical supervision (i.e., how and by whom?).
4. Student evaluation.
5. Job satisfaction of graduates.
6. Instructional methods.
7. Curriculum content.

8. Impact of graduates on employers, patients, and health care delivery.
9. Roles and functions of graduates in various settings.
10. Interdisciplinary teaching.
11. Comparison of primary care faculty with other nursing faculty.
12. Program costs.

RESEARCH IN CLINICAL PRACTICE

Primary care faculty have the advantage of constant contact with clinical agencies either with students or in their own practice. There are many researchable questions that arise about the care of patients —what is done, how it is done, and who does it. Only a small sample of possible topics can be listed here:

1. Patient outcomes with different providers.
2. Patient outcomes with different treatments or teaching methods.
3. Patient satisfaction.
4. Long-term effects of nurse practitioner care (i.e., functional status, days of hospitalization, morbidity).
5. Relationship of frequency of follow-up to outcomes.
6. Nurse practitioner-physician collaboration.
7. Cost of care using various providers and techniques.

It is much easier to get permission for a clinical study in an agency where the researcher is known, hence another advantage of researching in the practice setting. Often the research project results can be used to improve patient care or solve an administrative problem.

GETTING STARTED IN RESEARCH

A research project begins with a thought such as "I wonder which is better—," a dissatisfaction with the current status of teaching or practice, or a desire to describe a phenomenon. Through discussion and reading, a research question or hypothesis is formulated. A preliminary review of the literature will also reveal what is known about the subject.

From this point on, all but the most experienced researchers benefit from consultation in formulating a research design. It may be that the project is large enough and important enough to assemble a team. Too many nurses, perhaps trying to prove that they have the expertise, work in isolation. A mentor relationship with one or more experienced nurse colleagues or one in a related field is invaluable. Other health professionals can be consulted or perhaps become coinvestigators. Statistical consultation is also helpful although a nurse researcher should become generally familiar with the appropriate analytical methods for the particular design.

METHODOLOGY

The general categories of research designs that have been used most frequently are listed below (adapted from Isaac & Michael, 1971, p. 14).

1. *Historical* research reconstructs the past and often tests a hypothesis retrospectively.
2. *Descriptive* research describes a situation or area of interest.
3. *Developmental* research investigates patterns and sequences of growth or change over time.
4. *Case and field methods* study the background, current status, and environmental interactions of a given social unit.
5. *Correlational* research studies the extent to which one factor varies as a function of another.
6. *Causal-comparative or ex post facto* designs investigate possible cause-and-effect relationships by searching back through data retrospectively for plausible causal factors.
7. *Experimental* research investigates cause-and-effect relationships by exposing one or more experimental groups to one or more treatment conditions and comparing the results to one or more control groups (random assignment is a prerequisite).
8. *Quasi-experimental* design approximates the true experiment where it is not possible to control or manipulate variables. Groups are compared but there is no random assignment.

9.   *Action research* is designed to develop new skills and approaches to solving problems in an applied setting.

The methods listed above have been the mainstay of nurse researchers. However, a quiet revolution is taking place in behavioral fields that is having a "trickle-down" effect on nursing research. After wholeheartedly embracing the scientific method, that is, hypothesis-testing, researchers interested in the complexities of human behavior are warning of the "dangers of methodological transplant" (Engel & Filling, 1981, p. 14). The concern is that in controlling or ignoring a number of key variables there is a tendency toward isolated, microcosmic studies. Further, critics of the whole-sale application of laboratory methods to researching human experience believe methods that deal with simple and static events cannot be applied directly to complex, dynamic processes. The impact of the traditional scientific method, called the "received view" by its critics, is reviewed by Webster, Jacox, and Baldwin (1981). They lament the fact that nursing research and theory development has clung to the received view while other scientists have faced and accepted its limitations.

Hypothesis-generating methods

What, then, is the alternative? Engel and Filling (1981) suggest that more appropriate research strategies include observation, description, and interpretation. The researcher, without altering the environment, observes people (subjects) in their natural environment for long periods of time and describes behavior within the environment. This is the essence of the ethnographic or naturalistic method. Field and phenomenological research are also in this category of describing subjects in their natural surroundings rather than in the laboratory.

The inclusion of more descriptive methods in nursing research certainly is appropriate when studying nurses in expanded roles. It seems premature to compare the outcomes of care by nurse practitioners with that of other providers before there is a careful description of what each profession does given similar patient problems. It is unwise to test hypotheses before theory is developed about the phenomena being studied. Quantitative and some qualitative methods are suited to testing theory but are not as helpful in building theory. Qualitative methods such as the grounded theory approach proposed by Glaser and Strauss (1967) are finding many advocates in nurses who are interested in building nursing theory. The proponents of grounded theory emphasize the importance of generating hypotheses, concepts, and, eventually, theory from the data rather than fitting a "borrowed" theory to the data post hoc. Categories or their properties are developed from the data rather than measuring predetermined concepts. Since it appears that primary care nursing has little basis in existing theory, researchers would benefit from exploring some of these methods.

There is not room here to debate the virtues of quantitative versus qualitative methods extensively. The "truth" probably lies somewhere between the two. In fact, Gibbs (1979) suggests that hypothesis-generating and hypothesis-testing methods are complementary and necessary to move scientific knowledge forward. Ultimately, research questions arise from theory or practice and the best method should be chosen to answer the question. The potential teacher-researcher should become familiar with both categories of methods and choose those that will result in generating and testing new knowledge in primary care nursing.

DISSEMINATING THE FINDINGS

Often researchers do not let others know the results of their studies. This is particularly true of nonsignificant findings. However, research is wasted unless colleagues learn about it.

The first line of communication is in presentations at conferences where results can be quickly publicized. Even before the studies are complete, reporting progress is helpful to colleagues. Through these efforts, collaborative projects may result.

It is mandatory that the results of a study be reported to an agency or school where the data were gathered. The results can then be used in planning for better patient care or teaching.

Publishing results is more difficult and time-consuming. Some tips for getting articles published are:

1. Attend a workshop on writing and publishing.
2. Send query letters to journals to see if they are interested in the subject.
3. Find a mentor or more experienced colleague for consultation and moral support.
4. Write and rewrite.
5. Have your manuscript reviewed by several colleagues.
6. Rewrite paying attention to the journal's style sheet and reviewer's comments.
7. Submit it!

Even good research will not be published if the writing is poor. This is the reason collegial review is so important. Their critiques will be helpful because their perspective is more objective. If the contribution of colleagues is substantial, coauthorship can be offered. This kind of mentorship and networking will help achieve professional goals and upgrade nursing's academic standing.

If an article is rejected, the reviewer's comments can be used to rewrite and submit to another or the same journal. It is important to slant an article to the readership of a specific journal. The same study might be appropriate for either a nursing, educational, or medical journal if the introduction, results, and implications are written to the specific readership.

OTHER RESEARCH INVOLVEMENT

Not all teachers of primary care desire or need, for their professional existence, to do original research and to publish. However, there are other ways to support nursing research and advance teaching and practice. Other related activities are:

1. Read research articles.
2. Critique research articles.
3. Translate meaningful results into nursing care practices.
4. Utilize any single step in the research process such as developing a questionnaire.
5. Replicate a study.
6. Prepare a research grant proposal.

7. Coordinate a large research project.
8. Consult with other nurses who are doing research. (Sweeney, 1981, p. 117)

In some ways, the individual researcher or study is not important. It is only when the results are considered together with other knowledge that nursing as a profession is advanced. Similarly, primary care nursing and teaching will have a solid base as faculty conduct research and share their findings through presentations, publications, and application to their own practice.

REFERENCES

Engel, J. D. & Filling, C. M. Research approaches in health professions education. *Evaluation and the Health Professions*, 1981, *4*, 13–20.
Isaac, S. & Michael, W. B. *Handbook in research and evaluation.* San Diego: Edits Publishers, 1971.
Gibbs, J. C. The meaning of ecologically oriented inquiry in contemporary psychology. *American Psychologist*, 1979, *34*, (2), 127–140.
Glaser, B. G. & Strauss, A. L. *The discovery of grounded theory.* Chicago: Aldine Publishing Company, 1967.
Prescott, P. A. & Driscoll, L. Evaluating nurse practitioner performance. *Nurse Practitioner*, 1980, *5* (4), 28–32, 53.
Sweeney, M. A. Clinical nursing research: Exposing the myths. In J. C. McClosky & H. K. Grace (Eds.), *Current issues in nursing.* Boston: Blackwell Scientific Publications, Inc., 1981.
Webster, G., Jacox, A. K., & Baldwin, B. Nursing theory and the ghost of the received view. In J. C. McClosky & H. K. Grace (Eds.), *Current issues in nursing.* Boston: Blackwell Scientific Publications, Inc., 1981.

SUGGESTED READINGS

Cook, D. R. & LaFleur, M. K. *A guide to educational research*, 2nd ed. Boston: Allyn and Bacon, Inc., 1975.
Nachmias, D. & Nachmias, C. *Research methods in the social sciences.* New York: St. Martin's Press, 1970.
Oiler, C. The phenomenological approach in nursing research. *Nursing Research*, 1982, *31*, (3), 178–181.

Appendixes

Appendices

Appendix 1
Examples of Patient Write-ups

INITIAL DATA BASE

Chief Complaint. R. O. is a 24-year-old black, divorced woman who is referred from the city health clinic because of recurrent headaches.

History of Present Illness. Ms. O. believes the episodes began at age 12–13. The headaches are described as throbbing, in the occiput and both temples, and lasting 3–4 hours. They are always preceded by numbness, tingling, and weakness in one extremity, usually an arm. The paresthesias begin distally and progress proximally. Sometimes there are parethesias on the same side of the face as the affected extremity or visual disturbances described as blurring or areas blotted out by "shiny spots." This prodrome can last 45 minutes to an hour and infrequently occurs without a subsequent headache.

Episodes occurred at least twice a month for many years until 2 years ago when they began to occur almost weekly. Attacks do not seem to be related to time of day or any specific activity. They never occur during sleep. Aspirin does not relieve pain. Only effective palliative measure is lying quietly without head movement in a dark room.

Had an EEG 4–5 years ago that was negative. Taking combination birth control pills for 4 or 5 years.

Family History. Figure A 1-1 is the genogram for Ms. R. O.'s family. Denies any family history of diabetes, heart disease, cancer, tuberculosis, hypertension, arthritis, kidney disease, psychiatric disorders, or alcoholism. Son has allergies. Mother had "sick headaches" as a child.

Social History. Ms. O. is a housewife who lives with her parents, two younger sisters, and her two children in a 4-bedroom semi-detached house in the inner city. She was divorced two years ago and dates one man steadily. She is a high school graduate and works as a clerk in an insurance company. She sleeps 7–8 hours per night, neither smokes nor takes medication except for BCP (birth control pills). She drinks 1–2 alcoholic drinks on weekends. Her diet consists of coffee and toast for breakfast; a sandwich, soda, and potato chips for lunch; meat, a starch, and vegetable for dinner. She eats a candy bar daily.

Past Health History. Usual childhood diseases. Denies rheumatic fever. Had a concussion as a result of a fall when 7 years old, without

Figure A 1-1. Family History

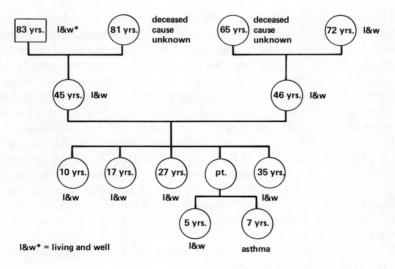

sequelae. Good health in adolescence. No hospital admissions except for childbirth.

Review of Systems

Skin: No history of rashes, pruritus, bruising, or other lesions.

Musculoskeletal: No history of fractures, weakness, myalgias, joint pain, heat redness, or swelling.

Lymph Nodes: No history of lymphadenopathy or pain.

Head: See HPI. No history of syncope or dizziness.

Eyes: Wears glasses for myopia. Last exam 6 months ago. No history of visual difficulties, diplopia, blurring, inflammation, except for scotoma during headache attacks.

Ears: Denies hearing problems, pain, discharge, tinnitus, or vertigo.

Nose, throat and respiratory: Infrequent colds. No history of sinusitis, nasal discharge, nosebleeds, hay fever, sore throat, tonsillitis, hoarseness, or cough. No asthma, fever, or night sweats.

Breasts: Breast-fed children for 3 months each. Denies trauma, lumps, pain, or discharge. Examines breasts irregularly, about 4–5 times per year.

Cardiovascular: No history of chest pain, palpitations, dyspnea on effort, paroxysmal dyspnea, fatigue, orthopnea, edema, cyanosis, hypertension. States that "blood fat" was elevated one year ago.

Gastrointestinal: Good appetite. No food intolerance. Teeth in good condition. Denies history of dysphagia, nausea, vomiting, hematemesis, indigestion, abdominal pain or discomfort, jaundice, or hepatitis. Has soft, brown stool every 1–2 days. Does not use laxatives.

Genitourinary: Treated for monilial vaginitis twice in last year. Denies history of venereal disease, dysuria, polyuria, nocturia, hematuria, frequency, urgency, or pain. Menses at 12. Menses regular every 24–26 days without dysmenorrhea or bleeding between periods. LMP (last menstrual period) 6 days ago. Three pregnancies, two full-term, uncomplicated deliveries, one spontaneous abortion at 6 weeks gestation. BCP for 4 years. Monitored every 6 months at city health clinics, states sexual relationship is satisfactory with boyfriend.

Endocrine: No recent changes in appetite, weight, activity, or heat tolerance. No history of polyphagia, polyuria or polydipsia.

Allergies: No known allergies or sensitivities to foods, drugs, pollens, or animals. Denies any history of hay fever or asthma.

Nervous System: *Motor:* Denies any problems with coordination, paralysis, muscle atrophy, or gait. *Sensory:* Denies paresthesias or loss of sensation.

Psychiatric: Considers self well-adjusted. No history of treatment of mental illness. Sleeps well. States that she has many friends and enjoys her job.

Physical Examination

Vital Signs: TPR–98^6–72–16, weight 130 lbs., height 5'4".

BP	Right	Left
Sitting	110/78	108/80
Supine	108/76	110/76
Standing	112/80	114/82

General Appearance: Alert, cooperative woman in no apparent distress.

Head: Normocephalic, symmetrical. No tenderness or masses.

Eyes: Wearing glasses. Tests 20/20 with glasses, 20/200 in each eye without. EOMs (extraocular movements) intact. No edema, ptosis, lid lag, jaundice. Sclera clear. Visual fields intact. PERRLA (pupils equal, round, and reactive to light and accommodation). A-V (arterial/venous) ratio 3:4. No retinal exudates or hemorrhages. Discs well-marginated.

Nose: No discharge. Septum in midline. No sinus tenderness.

Ears: No discharge. Canals clear. TM's (tympanic membranes) clear, pearly gray, with landmarks well visualized. Air and bone conduction normal. Hearing normal by whisper test.

Mouth: Teeth intact with 2 probable caries. No buccal lesions or gingivitis.

Throat: No exudates or lesions. Tonsils present but small.

Neck: No lymphadenopathy. Thyroid not palpable. No tenderness or masses. No bruits. Carotids 2+.

Cardiovascular: *Peripheral vascular:* Radial, popliteal, temporal, and dorsalis pedal pulses 2+. No vericosities.

Heart: PMI (point of maximal intensity) at 5th ICS (intercoastal space) at MCL (mid-clavicular line). No thrills or heaves. Apical rate 76, rhythm regular. No murmurs.

Chest: Symmetrical. Adequate respiratory expansion. No dyspnea. Tactile fremitus and vocal resonance normal. Chest clear to percussion and auscultation. No adventitious sounds.

Breasts: No lumps, tenderness, or discharge.

Abdomen: Soft, without masses or tenderness to deep or light palpitation. Bowel sounds normal in all quandrants.

Extremities: Color and temperature normal. No deformities.

Integument: Skin without lesions or significant scars. Nails and hair normal for age.

Musculoskeletal: No spine tenderness or deformity. All joints have normal range of motion without pain, heat, redness, or swelling. Muscle mass, strength, and symmetry normal for age and sex.

Genitalia: *External:* No lesions or swelling. No discharge. *Internal:* No vaginal lesions. Cervix nontender without lesions or discharge. Uterus and adnexa nontender, no masses felt.

Rectal: No hemorrhoids or fissures. Good sphincter tone. No tenderness or masses. Hematest negative.

Neurological: Judgment, orientation, and memory intact. Affect appropriate. Cranial nerves II-XII intact. DTR's (deep tendon reflexes) 2+. No Babinski. Motor: Posture and gait normal. Sensory: Superficial touch and dull-sharp sensation present and equal bilaterally. Cerebellar: Romberg negative, able to perform rapid alternating movements.

Problem List

1. Recurring headaches
2. Taking birth control pills
3. Possible elevated serum cholesterol

Initial Plan

1. Recurring headaches
   Assessment: Probable migraine headaches
   Diagnostic: Keep headache log
   Treatment: Discontinue birth control pills. Cafergot 1 tablet at beginning of attack and 1 tablet every half hour until relieved.

Maximum of 6 tablets per attack and 10 per week. Return to clinic after next attack or in 3 weeks.

Patient Education: Information given on probable diagnosis.

2. Taking birth control pills

Assessment: Needs an alternate form of birth control since BCP may exacerbate migraines.

Treatment: Discontinue BCP at end of present cycle. Reappoint for diaphragm fitting in 2 weeks.

Patient Education: Discussed alternatives. Patient prefers diaphram. Reviewed use and precautions. Understands possible relationship of BCP to migraines.

3. Possible elevated serum cholesterol

Assessment: Same

Diagnosis: Serum cholesterol, triglycerides, and HDL. Patient to record one week's dietary intake to assess fat content.

Treatment: None at this time.

Patient Education: Explained purpose of test and possible consequences of high cholesterol.

4. Incomplete data base

Diagnosis: Urinalysis, Pap smear, PPD (purified protein derivative)

PEDIATRIC PATIENT

Chief Complaint. 19 months old, white girl brought into clinic by mother who states child has not been gaining weight.

History of Present Illness. There has been a gradual decrease in weight in proportion to height since birth when both were at the 95th percentile. Birth weight was 7 lb. 3 oz., height 21.5″. Child is cared for by a pediatrician, Dr. P. Child's interest in food is decreasing, according to mother. Has had little illness (see Past Medical History) except for anemia diagnosed 1 year ago and treated with ferrous sulfate 0.6 cc per day for 6 weeks. Following treatment hemoglobin was 11.8 g.

Past Medical History. Had a severe "cold" at 1 year treated with unknown antibiotic 14 days. Symptoms of congestion and bronchitis subsided. Had diarrhea for 3 days soon after treatment. Had a similar "cold" at 13½ months with same treatment and sequelae. No accidents or other illnesses.

Family History.   Mother is 24 years old and has frequent urinary tract infections, otherwise is in good health. Father is 25 years old and in good health. The paternal grandmother has cataracts. Maternal grandfather has hypertension and osteoarthritis in his hips. Other grandparents are living and well. No history of diabetes, allergies, asthma, kidney disease, mental illness, or tuberculosis.

Social History.   Patient lives with parents in a 3-bedroom suburban home with a large fenced yard. There are no siblings and none are planned. Father is employed full-time as a computer programmer. Mother recently returned to part-time evening work as a medical technologist. Father or next-door neighbor babysits while mother works. Grandparents visit frequently.

Growth and Development.   Sat at about 5 months, walked at 1 year. Said single words at 12–14 months. Not very shy of strangers but is slow to warm up. Sleeps 8–9 hours waking at 7 a.m. Takes a 2-hour afternoon nap. Mother considers her very active.

Eats one good meal a day of meat, vegetable, juice, and starch. Prefers spicy foods like tacos. Dislikes milk but will eat some cheese or yogurt. Snacks on juice, fruit, and crackers. Mother restricts snacks before meals. States child seems "too busy to eat" and doesn't eat much at one time. Takes Tri-vy-sol 0.6 daily.

Is being toilet trained with no problems. Has language for voiding and BM but often tells mother after the fact.

Health Maintenance.   Immunizations up-to-date. Tine was negative at 15 months. No visual or auditory screenings done although parents have not identified any problems. No lead screen.

Review of Systems
HEENT (head, eye, ear, nose, and throat):   No head trauma, earaches, or infections, no problems with visual or auditory acuity. No eye infections, sore throats, croup or hoarseness. Coryza x2 (see PMH).
Respiratory: No bronchitis, pneumonia, dyspnea.

Heart: No history of murmurs or extra sounds.

GI: Diarrhea x2 (see PMH). No food intolerances except for loose stools with too much fruit. No constipation or colic.

GU: No problems voiding. No vaginal discharge as neonate. No change in color of urine.

Musculoskeletal: No problems with coordination or movement.

Neurological: No tremors or seizures.

Physical Examination

VS—Temp.: 100.2 R. BP not taken. Height: 33″ (95th%). Weight: 22 lbs.

General Appearance: Tall, slender, active, pleasant, well-groomed child.

Head: No lumps, scars, or lesions. No seborrhea or vermin. Scalp clean.

Ears: Some cerumen on right. Landmarks clear on TM's. Light reflexes present bilaterally.

Eyes: EOM's and visual fields intact. No strabismus. Red reflexes bilaterally, PERRLA.

Nose: Pink mucosa. No swelling or discharge.

Mouth: 14 teeth without cavities. No mucosal lesions. Gag reflex present. Tongue in midline.

Throat: No exudates or swelling. No hypertrophy of tonsils.

Neck: Supple. No lymphadenopathy. Thyroid not palpable. Trachea in midline.

Chest: Resp 18/minute. Symmetrical with breathing. No retraction. Lungs clear to auscultation. No adventitious sounds.

Heart: Rate 96. S_1 and S_2 clear to auscultation. PMI 1 cm in diameter and 4 cm left of LLSB in the 4th ICS. No murmurs, clicks, or gallops. Fermoral pulses strong bilaterally.

Abdomen: No hepatomegaly or splenomegaly. No hernias, masses, adenopathy, scars, or lesions.

Genitals: No discharge. Clitoris adequate, no erythema or lesions.

Extremities: Good muscle tone, mass, and strength. Symmetrical in size and movement. No hip clicks. Legs are straight.

Musculoskeletal: Spine straight. No pain or restriction on joint movement. No muscle or bone tenderness.

Neurological: Well-coordinated. No rigidity or spasticity.

Denver Developmental: Level of achievement at 2+ years.

Problem List
1. Well-child health maintenance.

Initial Plan
1. Well-child health maintenance.
   Assessment: Well child, tall and slender, but within normal limits.
   Diagnosis: Return in 3 months for weight and height check, hematocrit (11.5 today), and lead screen.
   Treatment: None.
   Anticipatory Guidance: Regarding temper tantrums, decreased appetite as growth rate decreases, poisons, accidents, fears.

EPISODIC NOTES

Patient 1

Subjective. Three weeks ago patient (a 55-year-old male) noted onset of intermittent hematuria, frequency and urgency (3 times per hour), trouble starting stream, nocturia (many!). Saw Dr. B. and was given Azogantricin, 2 tablets every 4 hours and referred to a urologist. Two weeks ago hematuria had stopped. Still had trouble with starting stream and nocturia. States sonogram showed small cyst in right kidney. No treatment given and told to return in 1 year. Childhood history of similar symptoms. Mother told him he probably had "stones" but never sought care for it after symptoms cleared.

Objective. TPR 98^7–84–22. BP 140/98 rt., sitting, 146/94 rt., supine. *Abd.*: Traumatic scars over epigastrium (bayonet wounds). Liver percussion 11 cm in width. Nontender. Moderate CVA tenderness over right flank. None on left.

Assessment. Kidney stone and/or cyst.

Plan/Diagnosis. Urinalysis with culture and sensitivity, serum calcium, IVP.

Treatment. Bactrim, 2 tablets every 12 hours x 14 days pending result of C&S. Adequate fluid intake. Return 1 week or sooner if pain worsens. Strain all urine.

Patient Education. Reason for symptoms, treatment. Importance of straining urine, taking medications as directed. Signs and symptoms to report.

Patient 2

Subjective. A 21-year-old white woman noted onset of "cold" approximately two weeks ago with symptoms of nasal congestion, sneezing, cough productive of large amount of white to greenish thick mucous. One week ago patient noted onset of sharp, intermittent pain in the right upper back that radiated to the anterior chest. The pain is intensified by coughing or deep breathing. Took cold tablets for last week without relief. Denies history of asthma, pneumonia, tuberculosis, frequent colds, swollen glands. Smokes 1 pack of cigarettes/day for 5 years. Says she felt warm the last 3 days but did not take her temperature. Came to the office today because pain is not relieved.

Objective. TPR 102-100-24. BP 118/74. Does not seem to be in acute distress. HEENT: No sinus tenderness or lymphadenopathy. TM's clear without injection. Throat not injected but tonsils erythematous and slightly enlarged. Nasal mucosa pink, small amount of clear discharge. Expectorated small amount of thick yellow sputum. Respiratory: Good, symmetrical expansion. Does not have pain with normal breathing. Lungs clear to percussion but rhonchi heard throughout posterior fields bilaterally. No rales or wheezing.

Assessment. Probable bronchitis, rule out pneumonia.
Plan/Diagnosis. Chest x-ray today, C&S of sputum.

Treatment. Ampicillin 500 mg p.o. q.i.d. for 10 days. Increase fluid intake. Return in 3 weeks. Rest in bed until temperature is normal. Discontinue smoking.

Patient Education. Importance of taking full course of antibiotics as directed. Relationship of bronchitis and smoking.

Appendix 2
Audit Form

(for use in auditing episodic note written when a
new problem is initially evaluated)

<u>Subjective</u>: description of client's problem/concern

    CHARACTERISTICS
       (location, quality, quantity,
       radiation)   included   omitted

    COURSE
       (onset, duration, frequency,
       seq. of events, current   included   omitted
       status)

    PRECURSORS OR AGGRAVATORS
       (family history, life
       style, previous episodes)   included   omitted

    ASSOCIATED SYMPTOMS
       (presence or absence of)   included   omitted

    TREATMENTS OR ALLEVIATING
    FACTORS
       (prescribed or self-remedies)   included   omitted

    SEQUELAE
       (complications, altered
       life style)   included   omitted

<u>Objective</u>: includes physical exam and possibly office lab data

    Evaluated body systems reflecting
      specific complaint location   included   omitted

    Evaluated body systems that would
      reflect potential causation   included   omitted

    Evaluated body systems that would
      reflect potential complications   included   omitted

Assessment:

ANALYSIS OF PROBLEM (what it is or what it is not)	included	omitted
CAUSATION (identifies potential etiology)	included	omitted
SEVERITY (progression or complications)	included	omitted
SIGNIFICANCE OF PROBLEM **TO CLIENT** (impact on client as a person; cognitive, emotional)	included	omitted

Plan:

GOAL STATEMENT	included	omitted
DIAGNOSTIC TESTS	included	omitted
TREATMENT REGIMEN	included	omitted
DISPOSITION (time of next visit, f/u activity at next visit, any referral if indicated)	included	omitted

Used by permission of Judith Ryan and Arlene Butz © 1980

Appendix 3

Final Evaluation of
Clinical Experience*

Student   Date

Instructor   Patient's age and diagnosis:

Quality of Performance: Rate the student by circling the
appropriate #:

      0 = Not applicable   3 = Adequate, safe
      1 = Not done   4 = Skillful
      2 = Inadequate

GENERAL BEHAVIOR	QUALITY	COMMENTS ON PERFORMANCE
Completes history and exams for interim visit in 45 minutes	0 1 2 3 4	
Relates material to literature, states references	0 1 2 3 4	
VERBAL PRESENTATION ASSESSMENT (Hx & P.E.)		
Data has a time sequence	0 1 2 3 4	
Data has organization	0 1 2 3 4	

*Developed by the Pediatric Faculty of the Primary Care
Department, University of Maryland School of Nursing

GENERAL BEHAVIOR	QUALITY	COMMENTS ON PERFORMANCE
Data as specific as possible	0 1 2 3 4	
Presentation concise	0 1 2 3 4	
Relevant clues followed	0 1 2 3 4	
Developmental assessment included	0 1 2 3 4	
Primary health care provider identified	0 1 2 3 4	
Health maintenance and immunization status determined	0 1 2 3 4	
Relevant family history explored	0 1 2 3 4	
Relevant PMHx, including medication, dosage, surgery, illness	0 1 2 3 4	
Relevant physical findings described succinctly	0 1 2 3 4	
VERBAL PRESENTATION: ANALYSIS AND PROBLEM IDENTIFICATION		
Major problems stated	0 1 2 3 4	
Supporting data presented for major problems	0 1 2 3 4	
Differential diagnosis of physical and psychosocial areas considered	0 1 2 3 4	

GENERAL BEHAVIOR	QUALITY	COMMENTS ON PERFORMANCE
Rationale for differential diagnosis given	0 1 2 3 4	
Sets priorities	0 1 2 3 4	
Gives reasons for priorities	0 1 2 3 4	
States clearly when more information needed	0 1 2 3 4	
VERBAL PRESENTATION MANAGEMENT		
States lab studies and tests student would do	0 1 2 3 4	
States specific reasons for these studies	0 1 2 3 4	
Describes counseling to be done	0 1 2 3 4	
States medication and dosage (when required)	0 1 2 3 4	
Writes a prescription in proper form	0 1 2 3 4	
Describes actions and side effects of medications	0 1 2 3 4	
Includes plans for follow-up	0 1 2 3 4	

GENERAL BEHAVIOR	QUALITY	COMMENTS ON PERFORMANCE
VALIDATION		
History sampled by instructor correlates with student hx.	0 1 2 3 4	
Physical findings by instructor match student findings	0 1 2 3 4	
Diagnoses correlate with expected student information level	0 1 2 3 4	
Lab and X-ray studies correlate with expected student information level	0 1 2 3 4	
Counseling is correct information	0 1 2 3 4	
Counseling is at level of patient and/or parent(s)	0 1 2 3 4	
Questions of parent are answered	0 1 2 3 4	
Child is addressed during counseling if age appropriate	0 1 2 3 4	
Implements plan for studies and treatment when decisions made	0 1 2 3 4	
Utilizes clinic resources	0 1 2 3 4	
Asks questions when needed to clarify task	0 1 2 3 4	

GENERAL BEHAVIOR	QUALITY	COMMENTS ON PERFORMANCE
WRITE-UP		
Complete history stated	0 1 2 3 4	
Logical sequence	0 1 2 3 4	
Follows accepted format	0 1 2 3 4	
Concise (no longer than 2 pages, preferably 1 page)	0 1 2 3 4	
Problems clearly stated	0 1 2 3 4	
Associated management specific and complete	0 1 2 3 4	
Follow-up included	0 1 2 3 4	
Charting principles used, signatures readable	0 1 2 3 4	

Appendix 4
Evaluation of
Clinical Performance*

The purpose of this evaluation is to provide both a numerical and descriptive assessment of the student's ability to obtain an appropriate data base from the patient, formulate a problem list, and establish an appropriate plan of management for common adult health problems encountered in an ambulatory setting. The student should know his/her own limitations as a health care provider and also function as a patient advocate.

The student's performance for each of the categories listed below is rated using the following scoring system except where otherwise indicated:

N =   Not asked or no assessment.

1 =   Incomplete. Generally has about half of relevant data or less. Requires many cues or clues from the preceptor for direction.

2 =   Usually obtains most (70%) of the relevant data. Some cues or clues from preceptor necessary to provide direction.

3 =   Usually has almost all (85%) of the relevant data. Requires few cues or clues from the preceptor.

4 =   Thorough and complete with little or no prompting from the preceptor.

*Developed by the Primary Care Department faculty at the University of Maryland School of Nursing for use in the Master's Program.

The chief complaint, HPI, review of systems, and patient profile are worth a total of 15%.

Chief Complaint

1. States reason for visit in
   patient's words.   N 1 2 3 4
2. States duration of problem.   N 1 2 3 4
3. Includes vital statistics –
   age, sex, race.   N 1 2 3 4
4. Identifies risk factors based
   on age, sex, race.   N 1 2 3 4

History of Present Illness

1. Describes onset of problem.   N 1 2 3 4
2. Describes course or progression
   of the problem.   N 1 2 3 4
3. Describes an episode (or the episode).   N 1 2 3 4
4. Describes current status of problem.   N 1 2 3 4
5. Identifies aggravating or
   alleviating events.   N 1 2 3 4
6. Identifies absence or presence
   of relevant past family history.   N 1 2 3 4
7. Identifies positive and negative
   response to appropriate
   associated symptoms.   N 1 2 3 4

Review of Systems

1. Screens appropriately for
   coexisting health problems.   N 1 2 3 4
2. Gives concise description for
   positive responses (including
   frequency, duration, and
   course/episode).   N 1 2 3 4
3. Identifes appropriate negatives
   for age, sex, race as well as for
   coexisting problems.   N 1 2 3 4

Patient Profile

1. Identifies social/occupational
   educational history.   N 1 2 3 4
2. Identifies activities of daily life.   N 1 2 3 4
3. Identifies family health history.   N 1 2 3 4
4. Identifies past health history.   N 1 2 3 4

<u>Physical Examination</u> – 25%

A. 1. Identifies expected findings
based on history.   N 1 2 3 4
2. Identifies actual normal
and abnormal findings.   N 1 2 3 4
3. Relates abnormal findings
to history.   N 1 2 3 4

B. <u>Technical Skills of Physical Examination</u>

1. Organized in performing inspection,
palpation, percussion, auscultation   N 1 2 3 4
(as relevant).
2. Discriminates between screening
evaluation and thorough evaluation   N 1 2 3 4
when indicated.
3. Exam is complete.   N 1 2 3 4
4. Evaluates accuracy and replication
of physical findings on the following
(circle one).

   a. Most obvious and some subtle findings
      usually correctly identified and examined.
   b. Usually all obvious and most (70%) subtle
      findings correctly identified and examined.
   c. Usually all obvious and almost all (85%)
      subtle findings correctly identified and
      examined.
   d. Usually all findings correctly and thoroughly
      identified and examined; does not interpret
      normal findings as abnormal or vice versa.

<u>Problem List (Circle One)</u>

1. Usually about half of abnormal findings omitted from list
   entirely.
2. Usually most (70%) abnormal data represented in some
   way.
3. Usually almost all (85%) of abnormal data represented in
   some way; listed in order of priority.
4. Usually separate manifestations are combined appropriately
   into problems and in priority.

Problem Assessment (Circle One)

1. Limited in ability to consider rule-outs for most problems. Sketchy in depth of understanding of problems.
2. Reasonably relates historical and physical data to determine rule-outs for <u>most</u> problems. May not exploit data fully (is overly cautious) or may make conclusions beyond the data (over interprets).
3. Reasonably relates data to determine rule-outs for <u>each</u> problem. Occasionally data may be over- or under-interpreted.
4. Evaluation of problems is thorough with consideration of appropriate rule-outs for each. Data not over- or under-interpreted.

Initial Plan (Circle One)

1. Most diagnostic tests during therapy or patient education for problems inappropriate (erroneous).
2. Includes some possible diagnostic tests, potential drug therapy, and patient education for each major problem with rationale.
3. Includes some possible diagnostic tests, potential drug therapy, and relevant patient education for each major and some minor problems with rationale. Identifies a goal for major problems.
4. Identifies goals for each problem and is thoroughly appropriate in suggested diagnostic tests, potential drug therapy, and patient education for each major and minor problem.

Adequacy of Knowledge Base

1. Demonstrates a sound knowledge of normal function of body system(s) involved in patient's health problem(s).   N 1 2 3 4

2. Demonstrates a sound knowledge of pathophysiology of body system(s) involved in patient's health problem(s).   N 1 2 3 4

3. Explains pathophysiology responsible for abnormal portions of the physical examination.   N 1 2 3 4

Rapport (Circle One)

1. Gaps in communication with patient. Is at odds with patient.
2. Listens and communicates concern for patient.
3. Relates to patient feelings and is supportive. Patient advocate.
4. Puts patients at ease, is supportive, concerned, and reassuring to patient. Is patient advocate.

Knowledge of Strengths and Limitations (Circle One)

1. Seems overly secure or insecure. Is hesitant or responds negatively to suggestions/criticisms.
2. Can articulate most strengths and limitations of capabilities. Is somewhat hesitant or insecure.
3. Knows strengths and limitations, is comfortable with self, responds positively to suggestions and criticism.
4. Is poised and articulate regarding own strengths and limitations and is very self-directed.

Oral Presentation (Circle One)

1. Presentation rambles in a nonpredictable manner. Somewhat coherent.
2. Most of presentation is logical and coherent.
3. Entire presentation is logically organized in a coherent manner but could be more concise.
4. Entire presentation is readily coherent and organized in a logical, concise manner.

Index

Index